Gluten-Free Dining in Seattle

BY ANDREA BIJOU

First Edition
First Printing, 2014

Cover design and page layout by maoStudios.
www.maostudios.com

ISBN-13: 978-0-615-89407-2

Yoj Creative
844 NE 92nd St
Seattle, WA 98115
www.yojcreative.com

Printed in the United States of America

Table of Contents

INDEX

PART 1: OVERVIEW

Seattle Rains Good Food & Progress

The moment you step into Seattle's green cornucopia you can feel it's a special kind of place. Even if you have lived in the green plateaus of this city your whole life, you know, there are not many places like it.

The air is fresh and crisp from the tall Evergreen trees decorating the city's parameter. A hike awaits you around every corner in one of Seattle's myriad of parks, while the mountains are only a half an hour drive away.

The people are weird. Like super weird. More on the introverted side, style is a bit elusive to these eccentric techies. It's not uncommon to see purple hair, Utilikilts and tattooed sleeves all on the same person.

Seattle is a green city. The people drive electric-powered, smart cars and biodiesel-fueled vehicles. Gardens and pea patches are common. Composting is encouraged and if you don't use your compostable garbage, the city collects it, breaks it down, and sells it for agriculture.

People drive slower, talk slower and generally live slower-paced lives. It's part of the culture of the West Coast to spend a good deal of time relaxing and enjoying the many fruits Seattle has to offer.

Last December, Seattle legalized marijuana. Soon, you will find marijuana cigarettes and other "green" goods sold alongside tobacco and alcohol. Washington is one of the few states in the entire United States that sells Marijuana legally. Could we be the next Amsterdam perhaps?

Most importantly, Seattle offers some of the best food on the Pacific. City officials allow food trucks to set up shop at any location around the city. So now you can find a fancy Cuban Fusion food truck right next to a Tom Douglas restaurant.

Seattle's food is expansive and continues to grow. Restaurants serve everything from American, American New, Cuban, Oaxacan, Family-Style Mexican, Thai, Vietnamese, BBQ, Korean, breakfast and brunch, café-style, to desserts and the list goes on. What's better about most of these restaurants? Many serve gluten-free options, whether the gluten is taken out or replaced with a delicious substitute.

This book is meant to serve as a guide for visitors and residents alike. I have been on a gluten-free hunt for over eight years and now I am giving you the skinny on what Seattle restaurants are cooking up for gluten-free customers. This book is organized by neighborhood and cuisine to serve as an easy restaurant guide for both locals and tourists.

Want to know what areas are best to stay or live in if you are gluten-free? Check out our neighborhood guide for the highest number of listings and ratings.

Traveling Gluten-Free

I didn't know much until I traveled. For example, did you know Denmark's housing rarely contains a bathtub? The porcelain rarities cannot be found in 90% of apartments in the city. Instead, Danish bathrooms consist of a shower head right above the toilet or a regular stand-up shower.

In the northern part of Norway, where the sun never shines, gluten allergies are a part of life and fully supported by the community. I was shocked to discover an entire section of a grocery store dedicated to gluten-free in a small village of 800 people in a Norwegian fjord.

Traveling is one of those off-campus universities that educates you through observing other cultures and adjusting to the cultural differences. I love to explore other cities and countries, it's what I live for. That said, traveling can cause a few serious setbacks for a person with gluten allergies.

Because I travel so often, I've developed a fool-proof list of tips that will help you get through the worst of it when you are out of your comfort-zone. This book is meant to make it easier to visit Seattle, but until there are more guidebooks for every area in the world, following your own tried and true methods will have to do.

1) Hotels. Don't stay in them. If you can, stay in a condo or a hotel with a kitchen. This will make your visit far easier. When you stay in a typical hotel, not only does it cost a lot more, you are also forced to eat out for every meal. When you eat out, you run the risk of eating more gluten, but also spend most of your time just looking for a place to eat. That process can suck up your vacation time, budget, and cause cranky spats with travel companions.

2) Snacks. Pack them in your luggage, your carry-on bags and your purse. Always have gluten-free snacks available along with water. Traveling is hard on your body, you are most often jet lagged, lost and not always sure when you will eat next. I recommend packing trail mix, jerky, gluten-free crackers, cheese, veggies and anything else that is low sugar and easy to carry.

3) Research. If you are visiting a country that speaks your native language, it's helpful to search online for a list of places to eat, grocery stores and vendors that carry or make gluten-free food. Better yet, map your dining experiences around where you are staying. I have recommended which neighborhoods are best for gluten-free in our neighborhood guide.

4) Foreign Travel. If you are traveling to an area that speaks another language and know very little of that language, learn a few common phrases, but most importantly learn how to say "gluten-free." In French it is "sans gluten" or "Je suis allergique au gluten." In Spanish it's "sin gluten." You get the idea. Look for these words on gluten-free products in grocery stores and mention it to your server. Most European countries are very familiar with gluten allergies.

5) Don't be Afraid to Ask. It's pretty easy to eat almost anywhere. Most dishes can be made without gluten. Just ask!

OVERVIEW

Representative Icons

Accompanying each listing in this book you will notice a number of icons. The meaning of each is defined below.

Represents how "gluten-free friendly" I find the restaurant to be, on a scale of one to five.

Helpful info about the restaurant, such as the primary focus and whether the location is a dedicated gluten-free facility or not.

Location address info.

Location phone number.

Website URL.

PART 2: BEST OF SEATTLE

Best Bakeries, Restaurants and Products

8 years ago eating gluten-free meant you ate cardboard and rock-textured baked goods. Eating out was often an unpleasant experience resulting in quizzical looks from wait staff when asked for gluten-free options. A salad or starvation were the go-to choices.

Those days are long gone, at least in Seattle. Pastry chefs, restaurants, bakers and product manufacturers alike have mastered the art (and challenge) of gluten-free food. In fact, some gluten-free pastries, cupcakes, and other desserts are better than the real thing.

My 'best of' section features the best of the best. I highlight the businesses who go above and beyond, ultimately making it much easier and delicious to eat with a gluten allergy.

Capitol Cider

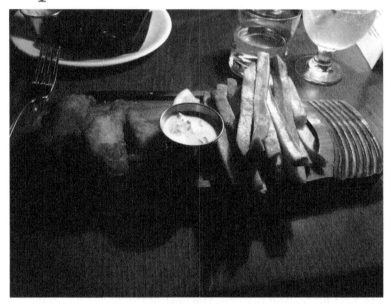

CAPITOL CIDER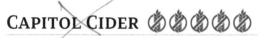

(i) *Gluten-Free Pub*
   Dedicated Gluten-Free

📍 **Address:**
   818 E Pike St
   Seattle, WA 98122

📞 **(206) 397-3564**

🔗 www.seattleciderbar.com

small portions
Dab didn't like

dont like location

"Pass me a pint you patsy, Mona's giving me the one eye..." and a lot to think about. Capitol Cider is one of those dark, old-boy bars commonly found near the Hill in D.C. I can see politicians engaging in rhetoric over a scotch and stogey. Complete with classical art and tall, Mahogany booths, visitors would never dedect that there is something radically different than its counterparts.

What's so unique about Capitol Cider? The entire kitchen is gluten-free. Do you know how hard that is to pull off for a bar? Admitttedly, they are a bit higher-end than a bar. The menu is more along the lines of American New or New Bar. Everything on the menu is gluten-free, from the fish and chips to the gnocchi. You can also order from an extensive menu of Ciders, with way too many options, which are also naturally gluten-free.

brunch sat & sun 10-3
happy hour m-Th 4-6
s-Th 10pm 12am

Late night 10-12 everynight
lunch 11-2

BEST OF SEATTLE

Jodee's Desserts

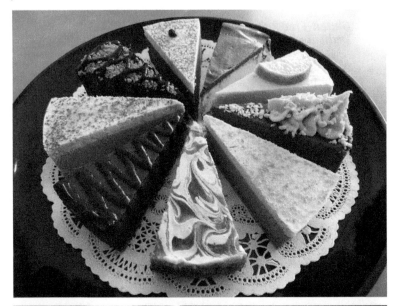

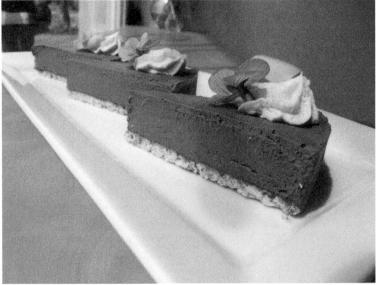

Photos provided by Jodee's Desserts

JODEE'S DESSERTS 🌾🌾🌾🌾🌾

ⓘ *Raw Desserts*
Dedicated Facility

📍 **Address** (*Green Lake*):
7214 Woodlawn Avenue NE
Seattle, WA 98115

📞 **(206) 525-2900**

🔗 www.jodeesdesserts.com

You can never have too much pie, especially at Jodee's. Made completely vegan out of coconut, fruits, nuts and veggies, Jodee's pies are a raw, gluten-free treat you cannot miss.

My favorite pie flavors are the carrot cake, pumpkin pie, key lime pie, banana cream pie, and tiramisu. They also carry chocolate mousse pie, chocolate cherry pie, chocolate malt pie, pecan praline pie, peppermint patty pie, and other seasonal flavors. This creative pie maker also serves smoothies, coffee, chocolates, and soups. The pie makers also supply pies to the local organic and natural grocery stores.

What's the best part about Jodee's desserts? No blood sugar blues. You aren't getting refined sugars or dairy in these treats just the best of what the earth makes naturally. As a part of a complete awareness to product purity, they use the Tensui Water Filtration System (www.TensuiWater.com) in all pie preparations. The pies are blended, without the need for baking, which sustains a nutritionally rich product.

Miro Tea

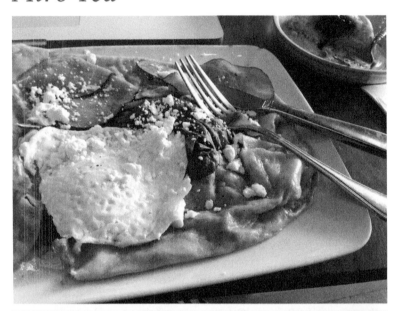

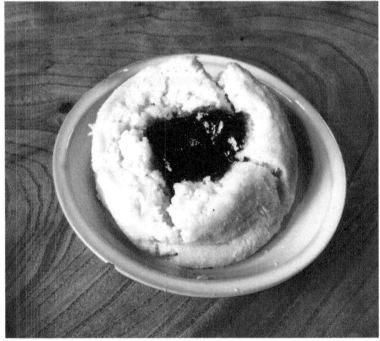

MIRO TEA

ⓘ *Tea Shop and Crêperie*
Not Dedicated Gluten-Free, but almost!

📍 **Address** *(Ballard)*:
5405 Ballard Ave NW
Seattle, WA 98117

📞 **(206) 782-6832**

🔗 www.mirotea.com

Don't let the hundreds of different teas fool you, Miro Tea is ample in gluten-free desserts and crêpes. Although I enjoy the myriad of tea options as well, which are blended for stress, calming, detox, energy, and a hundred other uses.

Miro Tea has replaced almost all of their baked goods and desserts with gluten-free options. I've seen the tea house carry gluten-free jam biscuits, lemon bars, banana bread, apple cake and carrot cake to name a few, not to mention their sweet and savory gluten-free crêpes.

It's hands down one of my favorite spots to read, write and enjoy a sugary treat.

BEST OF SEATTLE

Trophy Cupcakes

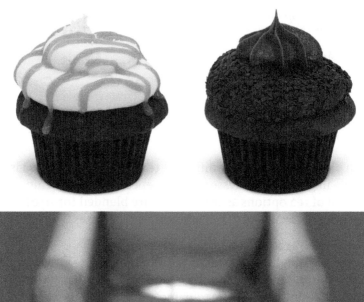

Photos provided by Trophy Cupcakes

TROPHY CUPCAKES

(i) *Cupcakes and Desserts*
     Not Dedicated Gluten-Free

(location) **Address** *(Multiple Locations)*:
            See page 105 for all locations.

(phone) **(425) 361-0033**

(link) www.trophycupcakes.com

Trophy Cupcakes is one of those cupcake makers who really got it right in the land of cakedom. Better yet, they have really amped up their street cred by offering 9 different gluten-free cupcake flavors.

What's 'right' about their sugary little treats? The cakes are moist and fluffy, while the frosting is tall and thick. Most notable are the completely unique designs, aka 'cake art.' If you follow Trophy on Facebook you will see what we are talking about. During Halloween, Trophy makes mummy, Frankenstein and pumpkin cupcakes. They even design for popular movies like "The Hunger Games", frosting flame and Mockingjay tops.

The Trophy bakers tested a gluten-free option for quite some time before releasing a suitable delicious gluten-free cupcake. They don't call themselves the magicians of mmm for nothing.

BEST OF SEATTLE

Café Piccolo

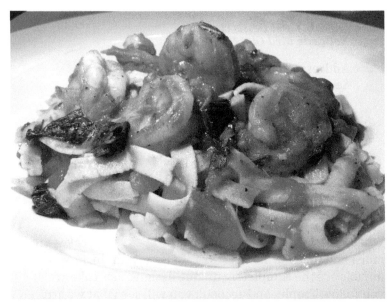

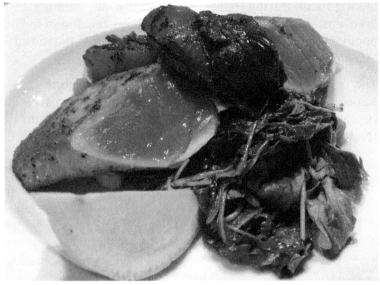

CAFÉ PICCOLO

ⓘ *Italian*
Not Dedicated Gluten-Free

📍 **Address** *(Maple Leaf)*:
9400 Roosevelt Way NE
Seattle, WA 98115

📞 **(206) 957-1333**

🔗 www.piccoloseattle.com

"When the moon hits your eyes like a big pizza-pie, that's amore." This song should cue every time a dinner guest walks through the front door of Café Piccolo. It's that kind of place. It's small, quaint and even displays a fishnet leg lamp in the back (full size of course).

Café Piccolo is a sweet little Italian restaurant, nestled in a residential area of Seattle called Maple Leaf. They serve gourmet (comfort) Italian food with gluten-free options for almost every dish.

When I first ate at Café Piccolo, they had a few gluten-free options like bread, fettuccine, and all the meat dishes could be made gluten-free. Now they can convert almost any dish.

What dishes are common on the menu? Lasagna, spaghetti, ravioli, fettuccine, breads, meat and veggies.

BEST OF SEATTLE

Homegrown

BEST OF SEATTLE

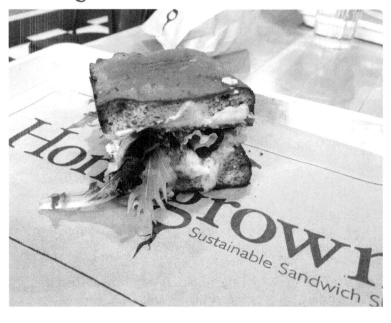

HOMEGROWN 🌾🌾🌾🌾

ⓘ *Sandwich and Soup Shop*
   Not Dedicated Gluten-Free

📍 **Address** *(Multiple Locations)*:
    See page 111 for all locations.

📞 **(206) 682-0935**

🔗 www.eathomegrown.com

When I say best, I mean THE BEST. Homegrown Sustainable Sandwich Shop is blowing my gluten-free mind, being one of the few shops in Seattle that makes gluten-free sandwiches for breakfast and lunch. Even better their sandwiches are damn good, in the I-want-to-eat-til-I-puke good.

Homegrown serves with a mission, "to create sandwiches out of sustainable ingredients but also to make sandwich creation sustainable itself." What does that mean exactly? Homegrown buys from local dairy producers, farmers and meat vendors. Everything is organic and free range. Homegrown also makes their own bread, in-house.

What kind of sandwiches do they serve? For breakfast they make a delicious bacon, egg & Beecher's cheese breakfast sandwich with garlic aioli. They also have a ham, cheese and egg sandwich, avocado and egg sandwich, lox and cream cheese and other items like oatmeal.

Lunch items include turkey, bacon and avocado, hummus and roasted peppers, roast pork, reuben revised, ham and cheese, squash, portobello and goat cheese. Not all together of course, but those items are just a sampling of what they offer.

Homegrown Sustainable Sandwich Shop has locations in Fremont, Capitol Hill and Queen Anne. I rank Homegrown as the best gluten-free sandwich shop in Seattle, so be sure to visit.

BEST OF SEATTLE

Portage Bay Cafe

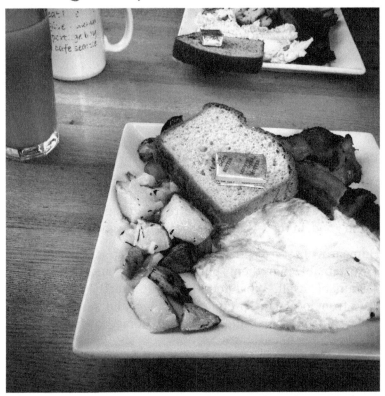

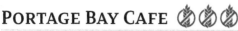

PORTAGE BAY CAFE 🌾🌾🌾

ⓘ *Breakfast and Lunch Cafe*
Not Dedicated Gluten-Free

📍 **Address** *(Multiple Locations)*:
See page 112 for all locations.

📞 **(206) 783-1547**

🔗 www.portagebaycafe.com

[handwritten notes: very good generous portions. Ballard location is nice because after you can walk around the locks]

See page 112 for all locations.

I can't get enough of Portage Bay Cafe and neither can anyone else apparently. That's why there is usually a long wait at all of their locations on a weekend morning. If you are willing to bare the 45+ minute wait you will be granted entrance into the best gluten-free cafe in Seattle. *[handwritten: make a reservation!]*

Everything there is handmade, organic and free-range. The gluten-free bread is moist and sliced thick. The pancakes are fluffy and stacked high. The fruit topping bar is constantly restocked for ample pancake and french toast devouring.

Portage Bay Cafe serves breakfast and lunch. They will make almost anything on the menu (and it is marked) gluten-free.

Portage Bay serves various egg and omelette breakfast dishes. You can also order gluten-free french toast and pancakes, along with sweet or savory porridge. For lunch choose from a variety of gluten-free sandwiches, burgers and salads.

BEST OF SEATTLE

Thrive

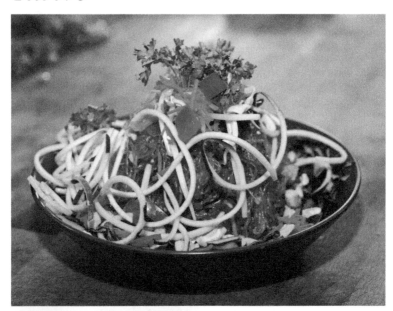

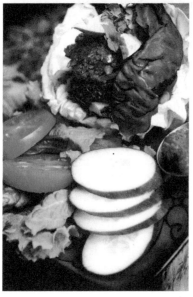

THRIVE 🌱🌱🌱🌱🌱

ⓘ *Raw, Vegan and Gluten-Free*
   Dedicated Gluten-free Facility

📍 **Address** (*Green Lake*):
   1026 NE 65th St
   Seattle, WA 98115

📞 **(206) 525-0300**

🔗 www.generationthrive.com

Thrive has me dancing a little hippy-dippy two-step. Not only is Thrive a gluten-free restaurant, they are also dairy-free, vegan, organic, low sugar, and try to buy local produce. I've recently started visiting Thrive for an afternoon vegetable juice, a feat they perfect, served up in a completely compostable plastic cup and straw.

Thrive will inspire you to cut out dairy because the food is so good without it. You would never know their dishes are dairy-free save for them telling you exactly what each dish doesn't have. Thrive also uses Agave nectar and other alternative sweeteners which score low on the glycemic index.

If you are looking for a healthy meal and education, Thrive is 'alternative diet central' station. The Buddha bowl and bella burger are my favorite lunch items.

BEST OF SEATTLE

Best Locally-Made Products

OLIVIA SUPERFREE

ⓘ *Wholesale breads, buns, pizza crusts, desserts.*
Dedicated Gluten-Free Facility

📍 **Address:**
2626 119th St SW A-3
Everett, WA 98204

📞 **(425) 267-2533**

🔗 www.oliviasuperfree.com

Sells wholesale to a large amount of restaurants, bakeries, and grocery stores in Seattle. Consider their products gluten, dairy, soy, rice, corn, potato, egg and peanut-free. You can purchase some of their products at PCC. Olivia Superfree was one of the first gluten-free bakers in Seattle, formerly known as Wheatless in Seattle.

ESSENTIAL BAKING COMPANY

ⓘ *Wholesale breads and buns.*
Not Dedicated Gluten-Free

📍 **Address:**
5601 1st Ave S
Seattle, WA 98108

📞 **(206) 545-3804**

🔗 www.essentialbaking.com

Wholesales nutty, gluten-free sandwich bread and buns to grocery stores in Seattle and also serves gluten-free sandwiches at their 4 café locations. This is the healthiest gluten-free bread you can get in Seattle. You can purchase Essential products at PCC, Whole Foods and other markets.

MANINIS GLUTEN-FREE

(i) *Wholesale breads, buns, flour mixes and pastas.*
Dedicated Gluten-Free Facility

📍 **Address:**
Seattle, WA

📞 **(206) 686-4600**

🔗 www.maninisglutenfree.wordpress.com

Wholesales to grocery stores and restaurants in WA, OR, CA, ID, HI and NY. In Seattle, you can purchase their products at PCC and Whole Foods. Maninis is a newer product manufacturer and has been all the rage for taste. Their products are practically indecipherable to gluten products.

NUFLOURS

(i) *Wholesale bread, cakes, pastries and treats.*
Dedicated Gluten-Free

📍 **Address:**
Seattle, WA

📞 **(206) 395-4623**

🔗 www.nuflours.com

Sells breads and desserts at the local farmer's markets in Seattle and wholesales to PCC. They have a good product, from rich brownies to crumbly cookies.

BEST OF SEATTLE

SKYDOTTIR COOKIES

ⓘ *Wholesale GF chocolate chip cookies*
Dedicated Gluten-Free Facility

📍 **Address:**
Ballard, WA

📞 **(206) 265-3195**

🔗 www.wp.skydottir.com

The best gluten-free old fashion chocolate chip cookies out there. Mostly sells wholesale, but you can order directly online. You can find their cookies at Whole Foods and many coffee shops around town.

TARTE NOUVEAU

ⓘ *Wholesale tarts and desserts*
Dedicated Gluten-Free

📍 **Address:**
Seattle, WA

📞 **(206) 524-3020**

🔗 www.tartenouveau.org

Gluten-free pastries made by a real pastry chef. Tarte Nouveau's desserts are fantastic. You can find Tarte Nouveau in the Amazon campus cafés in South Lake Union and in various other grocery stores. Contact directly for special orders.

PART 3: NEIGHBORHOOD GUIDE

Restaurants Listed by Neighborhood

Staying in a certain area of Seattle? We have listed out the best and most convenient places to dine by neighborhood. All neighborhood listings have a corresponding review in the Cuisine Guide section of this book.

You may notice some businesses who offer gluten-free are not featured. While I have tried to be as comprehensive as possible, I am not including everything and the kitchen sink. Gluten-free food is trending, which means some businesses have jumped on the bandwagon subtracting out gluten products to better serve the growing allergic community and we appreciate the effort. That doesn't mean the food is good and there aren't better places to eat. I am including most of my favorites (and some averages); places I have vetted, so you won't have a unpleasant experience.

As for Asian cuisine, there are too many to list. Let it be said, most restaurants serving Asian cuisine have many naturally gluten-free dishes if made without soy sauce. In this book, I am including my favorites; the Asian cuisine that stands out amongst the many.

NEIGHBORHOOD GUIDE

NEIGHBORHOOD GUIDE

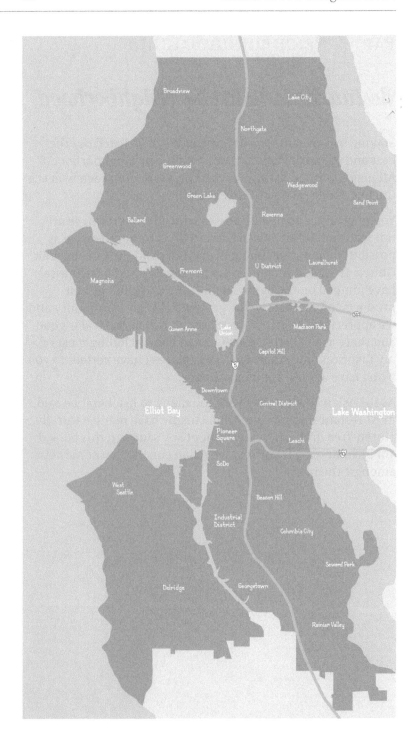

Ballard

Where the Norwegian fisherman settled, Ballard used to be a Fisherman's port, but now it's a hot spot for 30-somethings and for good reason. Some of the best restaurants and bars in Seattle are in Ballard. You won't find top-forty dance clubs here, although there might be a hidden dance club or two, it's mostly about beer and of course, good eating.

Ballard is well-known for small music venues, indie boutiques, sushi, and good ol-fashion debauchery.

Hipsters are abound, but more of a grown up hipster, dare we say yippie (yuppie-hippies)? So of course us "yippies" are catered to and provided gluten-free options.

There aren't a ton of hotel options, however airbnb.com can fix that problem.

Below are some of the best gluten-free restaurants in the Ballard area. Many have gluten-free bread options, pizzas, and desserts. The restaurants with three "no-wheat" symbols cater to gluten-free diners, but may only have one or two gluten-free alternatives.

NEIGHBORHOOD GUIDE

CUPCAKE ROYALE

ⓘ *Cupcakes and Desserts*
   Not Dedicated Gluten-Free

📍 **Address:**
   2052 NW Market St
   Seattle, WA 98107

📞 **(206) 883-7656**

🔗 www.cupcakeroyale.com

See full review on page 101.

FULL TILT ICE CREAM

ⓘ *Ice Cream and Pinball Arcade*
   Not Dedicated Gluten-Free

📍 **Address:**
   5453 Leary Ave NW
   Seattle, WA 98107

📞 **(206) 297-3000**

🔗 www.fulltilticecream.com/

See full review on page 120.

HOT CAKES MOLTEN CHOCOLATE

ⓘ *Desserts*
   Not Dedicated Gluten-Free

📍 **Address:**
   5427 Ballard Ave NW
   Seattle, WA 98107

📞 **(206) 420-3431**

🔗 www.getyourhotcakes.com

See full review on page 123.

NEIGHBORHOOD GUIDE

MATADOR

ⓘ *Tex-Mex Lunch and Dinner*
Not Dedicated Gluten-Free

📍 **Address:**
2221 NW Market St
Seattle, WA 98107

📞 **(206) 297-2855**

🔗 www.matadorseattle.com

See full review on page 140.

MIRO TEA

ⓘ *Tea Shop, Breakfast and Lunch Crêperie*
Not Dedicated Gluten-Free, but almost!

📍 **Address:**
5405 Ballard Ave NW
Seattle, WA 98117

📞 **(206) 782-6832**

🔗 www.mirotea.com

See full review on pages 15 and 124.

PALERMO RESTAURANT

ⓘ *Italian, Dinner*
Not Dedicated Gluten-Free

📍 **Address:**
2005 NW Market St
Seattle, WA 98107

📞 **(206) 297-2727**

🔗 www.palermorestaurant.com

See full review on page 144

NEIGHBORHOOD GUIDE

PORTAGE BAY CAFE 🌿🌿🌿🌿🌿

ⓘ *Breakfast and Lunch Cafe*
  Not Dedicated Gluten-Free

📍 **Address:**
  2821 NW Market St
  Seattle, WA 98107

📞 **(206) 783-1547**

🔗 www.portagebaycafe.com

See full review on page 22 and 111.

SHIKU SUSHI 🌿🌿🌿

ⓘ *Sushi*
  Not Dedicated Gluten-Free

📍 **Address:**
  5310 Ballard Ave NW
  Seattle, WA 98107

📞 **(206) 588-2151**

🔗 www.shikusushi.com

See full review on page 155.

THE HI-LIFE 🌿🌿🌿

ⓘ *American*
  Not Dedicated Gluten-Free

📍 **Address:**
  5425 Russell Ave NW
  Seattle, WA 98107

📞 **(206) 784-7272**

🔗 www.chowfoods.com/hi-life

See full review on page 96 and 112.

NEIGHBORHOOD GUIDE

TRADER JOE'S 🧅🧅🧅

ⓘ   *Natural Grocery Store*
    Not Dedicated Gluten-Free

📍 **Address:**
    4609 14th Ave NW
    Seattle, WA 98107

📞 **(206) 783-0498**

🔗 www.traderjoes.com

See full review on page 128.

Capitol Hill

Some of Seattle's most eccentric residents live in Capitol Hill. Known for being gay-friendly, tattooed and just plain old flamboyant (in an awesome kind-of way) the people of Capitol Hill are always up to give visitors a good show. If you are checking out this part of town, expect drama and drag queens around every corner.

Dance clubs are a plenty in this neighborhood and are some of the best in Seattle. Our Place, Havana and The Wild Rose are a few of our favorite site-seeing dance clubs.

You can also expect a lot of good food, because hey, queens have good taste. Don't judge a restaurant by its exterior, Capitol Hill has some of the most whimsical dining options from Speak Easy's requiring special codes for entry to basement Tibetan food.

Capitol Hill sits just up the hill from South Lake Union and the Downtown sector. Many visitors choose to stay in those areas because of the convenience, if you are, venture up to this area, but figure out where you are going first as to avoid walking around for hours in mayhem.

NEIGHBORHOOD GUIDE

Three "no-wheat" symbols or less means limited gluten-free options, however they still do a great job catering to gluten-free.

ANNAPURNA CAFE

ⓘ *Indian*
   Not Dedicated Gluten-Free

📍 **Address:**
   1833 Broadway
   Seattle, WA 98122

📞 **(206) 320-7770**

🔗 www.annapurnacafe.com

See full review on page 130.

8 OZ BURGER BAR

ⓘ *Burger Joint*
   Not Dedicated Gluten-Free

📍 **Address:**
   1401 Broadway
   Seattle, WA 98122

📞 **(206) 466-5989**

🔗 www.8ozburgerbar.com

See full review on page 113.

NEIGHBORHOOD GUIDE

BLUE MOON BURGERS

(i) *Burger Joint*
Not Dedicated Gluten-Free

📍 **Address:**
523 Broadway East
Seattle, WA 98102

📞 **(206) 325-2000**

🔗 www.bluemoonburgers.com

See full review on page 114.

CAPITOL CIDER

(i) *Gluten-Free Pub*
Dedicated Gluten-Free

📍 **Address:**
818 E Pike St
Seattle, WA 98122

📞 **(206) 397-3564**

🔗 www.seattleciderbar.com

See full review on page 11 and 92.

CUPCAKE ROYALE

(i) *Cupcakes and Desserts*
Not Dedicated Gluten-Free

📍 **Address:**
1111 East Pike St
Seattle, WA 98122

📞 **(206) 883-7656**

🔗 www.cupcakeroyale.com

See full review on page 101.

NEIGHBORHOOD GUIDE

GUILT FREE GOODNESS

ⓘ *Bakery*
Dedicated Gluten-Free

📍 **Address:**
219 Broadway E
Seattle, WA 98102

📞 **(360) 794-5266**

🔗 www.guilt-free-goodness.com

See full review on page 103.

HEALEO

ⓘ *Juice, Supplements, and Lunch*
Not Dedicated Gluten-Free

📍 **Address:**
1520 15th Ave
Seattle, WA 98122

📞 **(206) 453-5066**

🔗 www.healeo.com

See full review on page 148.

HOMEGROWN

ⓘ *Sandwich and Soup Shop*
Not Dedicated Gluten-Free

📍 **Address:**
1531 Melrose Ave
Seattle, WA 98122

📞 **(206) 682-0935**

🔗 www.eathomegrown.com

See full review on page 21 and 148.

NEIGHBORHOOD GUIDE

I ♥ My GFF 🌱🌱🌱🌱

(i) *Rice Bowls*
Dedicated Gluten-Free
Food Truck

Visit Website for Location.

🔗 www.ilovemygff.com

See full review on page 111.

Mamnoon 🌱🌱🌱

(i) *Middle Eastern, Mediterranean*
Not Dedicated Gluten-Free

📍 **Address:**
1508 Melrose Ave
Seattle, WA 98122

📞 **(206) 906-9606**

🔗 www.mamnoonrestaurant.com

See full review on page 137.

Palermo Restaurant 🌱🌱🌱🌱

(i) *Pizza and Italian*
Not Dedicated Gluten-Free

📍 **Address:**
350 15th Ave E
Seattle, WA 98112

📞 **(206) 322-3875**

🔗 www.palermorestaurant.com

See full review on page 144.

NEIGHBORHOOD GUIDE

PLUM BISTRO 🌱🌱🌱🌱

ⓘ *Raw and Vegan*
Not Dedicated Gluten-Free

📍 **Address:**
1429 12th Ave
Seattle, WA 98122

📞 **(206) 838-5333**

🔗 www.plumbistro.com

See full review on page 160.

REMEDY TEAS 🌱🌱🌱

ⓘ *Tea*
Not Dedicated Gluten-Free

📍 **Address:**
345 15th Ave E
Seattle, WA 98112

📞 **(206) 323-4832**

🔗 www.remedyteas.com

See full review on page 156.

TAYLOR SHELLFISH 🌱🌱🌱🌱

ⓘ *Seafood*
Not Dedicated Gluten-Free

📍 **Address:**
1521 Melrose Ave
Seattle, WA 98101

📞 **(206) 501-4321**

🔗 www.taylormelrose.com

See full review on page 153.

NEIGHBORHOOD GUIDE

TRADER JOE'S 🔥🔥🔥

ⓘ *Natural Grocery Store*
Not Dedicated Gluten-Free

📍 **Address:**
1700 Madison St
Seattle, WA 98122

📞 **(206) 322-7268**

🔗 www.traderjoes.com

See full review on page 128.

TERRA PLATA 🔥🔥🔥

ⓘ *Modern American*
Not Dedicated Gluten-Free

📍 **Address:**
1501 Melrose Ave
Seattle, WA 98122

📞 **(206) 325-1501**

🔗 www.terraplata.com

See full review on page 100.

ZAW 🔥🔥🔥

ⓘ *Artisan Pizza*
Not Dedicated Gluten-Free

📍 **Address:**
1424 E. Pine St
Seattle, WA 98122

📞 **(206) 325-5528**

🔗 www.zaw.com

See full review on page 146.

NEIGHBORHOOD GUIDE

Downtown

If you like the touristy side of travel, then downtown is probably where you will stay. Home to Pike Place Market, Pacific Place Mall, The Seattle Art Museum, and Pioneer Square, downtown is busy with tourists from allover the world.

Most of the city's hotels are in the downtown area, hence the spike in tourism in this area. It's also home to a plethora of dance clubs in Belltown and an active nightlife.

The Pink Door, Wasabi Bistro, Long Provincial, Icon Grill, Cyber Dogs, PF Chang's, Contigo, Biscuit Bitch and Andaluca are all located in the downtown sector.

Three "no-wheat" symbols or less means limited gluten-free options, however they still do a great job catering to gluten-free.

ANDALUCA 🌾🌾🌾

ⓘ *Mediterranean*
    Not Dedicated Gluten-Free

📍 **Address:**
    407 Olive Way
    Seattle, WA 98101

📞 **(206) 382-6999**

🔗 www.andaluca.com

See full review on page 136.

NEIGHBORHOOD GUIDE

BISCUIT BITCH 🌾🌾🌾

ⓘ *Comfort Food, Breakfast and Lunch*
Not Dedicated Gluten-Free

📍 **Address:**
1909 1st Ave
Seattle, WA 98101

📞 **(206) 441-7999**

🔗 www.biscuitbitch.com

See full review on page 91.

BOKA RESTAURANT & BAR 🌾🌾🌾

ⓘ *American New/Northwest*
Not Dedicated Gluten-Free

📍 **Address:**
1010 First Ave
Seattle, WA 98104

📞 **(206) 357-9000**

🔗 www.bokaseattle.com

See full review on page 97.

COFFEE &
A SPECIALTY BAKERY 🌾🌾🌾🌾🌾

ⓘ *Café and Bakery*
Dedicated Gluten-Free

📍 **Address:**
1500 Western Ave
Seattle, WA 98101

📞 **(206) 280-7946**

See full review on page 100.

NEIGHBORHOOD GUIDE

CHEESECAKE FACTORY

ⓘ *American*
  Not Dedicated Gluten-Free

📍 **Address:**
  700 Pike St
  Seattle, WA 98109

📞 **(206) 652-5400**

🔗 www.thecheesecakefactory.com

See full review on page 93.

CONTIGO

ⓘ *Modern Mexican*
  Not Dedicated Gluten-Free
  Food Truck

  Visit website for daily locations.

🔗 www.contigoseattle.com

See full review on page 138.

CYBER DOGS INTERNET CAFÉ

ⓘ *Vegetarian Hot Dogs*
  Not Dedicated Gluten-Free

📍 **Address:**
  909 Pike St
  Seattle, WA 98101

📞 **(206) 405-3647**

🔗 www.cyber-dogs.com

See full review on page 160.

NEIGHBORHOOD GUIDE

FRAN'S CHOCOLATES

(i) *Chocolatier*
Dedicated Gluten-Free

(location) **Address:**
1325 1st Ave
Seattle, WA 98101

(phone) **(206) 682-0168**

(link) www.franschocolates.com

See full review on page 120.

ICON GRILL

(i) *American*
Not Dedicated Gluten-Free

(location) **Address:**
1933 5th Ave
Seattle, WA 98101

(phone) **(206) 441-6330**

(link) www.icongrill.com

See full review on page 94.

MOD PIZZA

(i) *Pizza*
Not Dedicated Gluten-Free

(location) **Address:**
1302 6th Ave
Seattle, WA 98101

(phone) **(206) 332-0200**

(link) www.modpizza.com

See full review on page 143.

NEIGHBORHOOD GUIDE

TANGO RESTAURANT AND LOUNGE 🌾🌾🌾🌾

ⓘ *Spanish and Cuban Fusion*
Not Dedicated Gluten-Free

📍 **Address:**
1100 Pike St
Seattle, WA 98101

📞 **(206) 583-0382**

🔗 www.tangorestaurant.com

See full review on page 154.

THE JUICY CAFE 🌾🌾🌾

ⓘ *Breakfast and Juice Cafe, Vegetarian*
Not Dedicated Gluten-Free

📍 **Address:**
725 Pike St, Fl 2nd
Seattle, WA 98101

📞 **(206) 682-6960**

🔗 www.thejuicycafe.com

See full review on page 162.

THE PINK DOOR 🌾🌾

ⓘ *Italian*
Not Dedicated Gluten-Free

📍 **Address:**
1919 Post Alley
Seattle, Pike Place Market

📞 **(206) 443-3241**

🔗 www.thepinkdoor.net

See full review on page 134.

NEIGHBORHOOD GUIDE

TULIO RISTORANTE 🌾🌾🌾

ⓘ *Italian*
Not Dedicated Gluten-Free

📍 **Address:**
1100 5th Ave
Seattle, WA 98101

📞 **(206) 624-5500**

🔗 www.tulio.com

See full review on page 135.

WASABI BISTRO 🌾🌾🌾🌾🌾

ⓘ *Sushi*
Not Dedicated Gluten-Free

📍 **Address:**
2311 2nd Ave
Seattle, WA 98121

📞 **(206) 441-6044**

🔗 www.wasabiseattle.com

See full review on page 154.

Eastlake

Eastlake is a little nook near South Lake Union just before you reach the downtown area of Seattle. It's densely populated with condos, houses and several marinas. Parking is scarce, but there are a few little gems in this area that are worth checking out.

In the summer, Eastlake is a beautiful area to spend an afternoon lunching. Many of the restaurants have outdoor patios and stunning views of Lake Union.

NEIGHBORHOOD GUIDE

Three "no-wheat" symbols or less means limited gluten-free options, however they still do a great job catering to gluten-free.

EASTLAKE BAR AND GRILL 🌾🌾🌾

ⓘ   *Bar and Grill*
Not Dedicated Gluten-Free

📍   **Address:**
2947 Eastlake Ave E
Seattle, WA 98102

📞   **(206) 957-7777**

🔗   www.neighborhoodgrills.com

See full review on page 93.

LITTLE WATER CANTINA 🌾🌾🌾

ⓘ   *Mexican, Tacos*
Not Dedicated Gluten-Free

📍   **Address:**
2865 Eastlake Ave E
Seattle, WA 98102

📞   **(206) 397-4940**

🔗   www.littlewatercantina.com

See full review on page 140.

NEIGHBORHOOD GUIDE

Ravish

ⓘ *American New*
   Not Dedicated Gluten-Free

📍 **Address:**
   2956 Eastlake Ave E
   Seattle, WA 98102

📞 **(206) 913-2497**

🔗 www.ravishoneastlake.com

See full review on page 98.

Siam Thai Cuisine

ⓘ *Thai*
   Not Dedicated Gluten-Free

📍 **Address:**
   1629 Eastlake Ave E
   Seattle, WA 98102

📞 **(206) 322-6174**

🔗 www.siamthairestaurants.com

See full review on page 158.

Eastside

This book is mostly focused on gluten-free restaurants in Seattle proper, but since there are a few options on the eastside of Lake Washington (East of Seattle) some of the restaurants in this area are included.

The "Eastside" is comprised of Bellevue, Redmond, Kirkland, Woodinville and maybe Issaquah. All of these cities are a little different from each other, but are the same in that they lack Seattle's character and charm. Bellevue is a rich, high-rising

NEIGHBORHOOD GUIDE

mecca of pricey shopping centers and corporate blah-ness. Kirkland isn't high-rising, but is definitely very rich. The city sits on the shore front of Lake Washington and attracts an American Idol crowd. Woodinville and Redmond are wealthy areas too, but with a much thicker backdrop of woods. Microsoft has made a sprawling home in Redmond, so many of the folks who live in this area hail from the tech-giant. Woodinville is notable for wine and the one place on the eastside I recommend visiting during the summer for wine tasting and outdoor concerts.

In all honesty, the Eastside is not my favorite place. All the character and eccentricity you will find in Seattle proper, ceases to exist out east. The rich of the rich live in the east and unfortunately aren't always the most humblest of people. I try to stay on the westside if I can help it, however if I find myself out in these parts, it is nice to know where a few gluten-free options are.

Three "no-wheat" symbols or less means limited gluten-free options, however they still do a great job catering to gluten-free.

AUNT LOUISE'S SECRET

(i) *Bed and Breakfast*
     Not Dedicated Gluten-Free

Q   **Address:**
    14241 NE Woodinville-Duvall Rd #154
    Woodinville, WA 98072

☎   **(206) 351-8858**

🔗   www.auntlouisessecret.com

See full review on page 108.

See full review on page 108.

Cactus Restaurants

ⓘ *Southwestern and Mexican Cuisine*
Not Dedicated Gluten-Free

📍 **Bellevue:**
535 Bellevue Way SE
Bellevue, WA 98004

📞 **(425) 455-4321**

📍 **Kirkland:**
121 Park Ln
Kirkland, WA 98033

📞 **(425) 893-9799**

🔗 www.cactusrestaurants.com

See full review on page 138.

Canyons Restaurant

ⓘ *American*
Not Dedicated Gluten-Free

📍 **Address:**
15740 Redmond Way
Redmond, WA 98052

📞 **(425) 556-1390**

🔗 www.canyonsrestaurant.com

See full review on page 92.

Cupcake Royale

ⓘ *Cupcakes and Desserts*
Not Dedicated Gluten-Free

📍 **Address:**
21 Bellevue Way NE
Bellevue, WA 98004

📞 **(425) 454-7966**

🔗 www.cupcakeroyale.com

See full review on page 101.

NEIGHBORHOOD GUIDE

EDEN B BAKERY 🌾🌾🌾🌾

ⓘ *Bakery and Café*
Dedicated Gluten-Free

📍 **Address:**
120 116th Ave NE
Bellevue, WA 98004

📞 **(425) 462-2224**

🔗 www.edenbbakery.com

See full review on page 102.

ESSENTIAL BAKING COMPANY 🌾🌾🌾🌾🌾

ⓘ *Breakfast and Lunch Cafe*
Not Dedicated Gluten-Free

📍 **Address:**
990 102nd Avenue NE
Bellevue, WA 98004

📞 **(206) 876-3770**

🔗 www.essentialbaking.com

See full review on page 148.

FLYING APRON 🌾🌾🌾🌾🌾

ⓘ *Gluten-Free Bakery*
Dedicated Facility

📍 **Address:**
16541 Redmond Way, Ste E
Redmond, WA 98052

📞 **(206) 442-1115**

🔗 www.flyingapron.com

See full review on page 102.

Fran's Chocolates 🌾🌾🌾🌾🌾

ⓘ *Chocolatier*
Dedicated Gluten-Free

📍 **Address:**
10036 Main St
Seattle, WA 98004

📞 **(425) 453-1698**

🔗 www.franschocolates.com

See full review on page 147.

Garlic Jim's Famous Gourmet Pizza 🌾🌾🌾

ⓘ *Pizza Delivery*
Not Dedicated Gluten-Free

📍 **Bothell:**
18404 120th Ave NE
Bothell, WA 98011

📞 **(425) 483-5555**

📍 **Kirkland:**
9758 NE 119th Way
Kirkland, WA 98034

📞 **(425) 307-1122**

📍 **Kirkland:**
8431 122nd Ave NE
Kirkland, WA 98033

📞 **(425) 822-8881**

📍 **Redmond:**
11523 Avondale Rd NE
Redmond, WA 98052

📞 **(425) 861-9000**

🔗 www.garlicjims.com

See full review on page 142.

NEIGHBORHOOD GUIDE

I ♥ My GFF 🌾🌾🌾🌾🌾

(i) *Rice Bowls*
Dedicated Gluten-Free
Food Truck

Visit Website for Location.

🔗 www.ilovemygff.com

See full review on page 111.

Matador 🌾🌾🌾

(i) *Tex-Mex*
Not Dedicated Gluten-Free

📍 **Address:**
7824 Leary Way NE
Redmond, WA 98052

📞 **(425) 883-2855**

🔗 www.matadorseattle.com

See full review on page 140.

Meritage Meadows Inn 🌾🌾🌾🌾🌾

(i) *Bed and Breakfast*
Not Dedicated Gluten-Free

📍 **Address:**
21407 NE Union Hill Rd
Redmond, WA 98053

📞 **(425) 487-4019**

🔗 www.meritagemeadows.com

See full review on page 108.

NEIGHBORHOOD GUIDE

MOD PIZZA 🌾🌾

ⓘ *Pizza*
Not Dedicated Gluten-Free

📍 **Bellevue:**
317 Bellevue Way NE
Bellevue, WA 98004

📞 **(425) 455-0141**

📍 **Redmond:**
8900 161st Ave NE
Redmond, WA 98052

📞 **(425) 497-5104**

🔗 www.modpizza.com

See full review on page 143.

PCC NATURAL MARKETS 🌾🌾🌾🌾🌾

ⓘ *Natural and Organic Grocery Store*
Not Dedicated Gluten-Free

📍 **Issaquah:**
Pickering Place
1810 12th Ave NW
Issaquah, WA 98027

📞 **(425) 369-1222**

📍 **Kirkland:**
10718 NE 68th
Kirkland, WA 98033

📞 **(425) 828-4622**

📍 **Redmond:**
11435 Avondale Rd NE
Redmond, WA 98052

📞 **(425) 285-1400**

🔗 www.pccnaturalmarkets.com

See full review on page 127.

NEIGHBORHOOD GUIDE

PF CHANG'S

ⓘ *Chinese*
Not Dedicated Gluten-Free

📍 **Address:**
Bellevue Square
525 Bellevue Square
Bellevue, WA 98004

📞 **(425) 637-3582**

🔗 www.pfchangs.com

See full review on page 117.

ROMIO'S PIZZA

ⓘ *Pizza Parlor*
Not Dedicated Gluten-Free

📍 **Factoria:**
3615 Factoria Blvd SE
Bellevue, WA 98006

📞 **(425) 747-3000**

📍 **Kirkland:**
11422 NE 124th St
Kirkland, WA 98034

📞 **(425) 820-3300**

🔗 www.romiospizzafactoria.com

🔗 www.romioskirkland.com

See full review on page 145.

NEIGHBORHOOD GUIDE

SAGE'S RESTAURANT 🌾🌾

ⓘ *Italian*
   Not Dedicated Gluten-Free

📍 **Address:**
   15916 NE 83rd Street
   Redmond, WA 98052

📞 **(425) 881-5004**

🔗 www.sagesrestaurant.com

See full review on page 134.

SEASTAR RESTAURANT AND RAW BAR 🌾🌾🌾

ⓘ *Seafood*
   Not Dedicated Gluten-Free

📍 **Address:**
   205 108th Ave NE
   Bellevue, WA 98004

📞 **(425) 456-0010**

🔗 www.seastarrestaurant.com

See full review on page 152.

SWEET CAKES BAKERY 🌾🌾🌾🌾

ⓘ *Desserts*
   Dedicated Facility

📍 **Address:**
   128 Park Lane
   Kirkland, WA 98033

📞 **(425) 821-6565**

🔗 www.sweetcakeskirkland.com

See full review on page 104.

NEIGHBORHOOD GUIDE

TRADER JOE'S 🔥🔥🔥

ⓘ *Natural Grocery Store*
Not Dedicated Gluten-Free

📍 **Bellevue:**
15563 NE 24th ST
Bellevue, WA 98007

📞 **(425) 641-5069**

📍 **Redmond:**
15932 Redmond Way
Redmond, WA 98052

📞 **(425) 883-1624**

📍 **Kirkland:**
12632 120th Ave NE
Kirkland, WA 98034

📞 **(425) 823-1685**

🔗 www.traderjoes.com

See full review on page 128.

TROPHY CUPCAKES 🔥🔥🔥🔥

ⓘ *Cupcakes and Desserts*
Not Dedicated Gluten-Free

📍 **Address:**
700 110th Ave NE #260
Bellevue, WA 98004

📞 **(425) 361-0033**

🔗 www.trophycupcakes.com

See full review on page 17 and 104.

WHOLE FOODS MARKETS 🌾🌾🌾🌾🌾

ⓘ *Natural Grocery Store*
   Not Dedicated Gluten-Free

📍 **Bellevue:**   📍 **Redmond:**
   888 116th Ave NE   17991 Redmond Way
   Bellevue, WA 98004   Redmond, WA 98052

📞 **(425) 462-1400**   📞 **(425) 881-2600**

🔗 www.wholefoodsmarket.com

See full review on page 129.

Fremont

Oh Fremont how I love thee. I solved your troll's riddle and am happy as can be to frolic in your landscape of peace and happiness. Have I clued you into the vibe of this Utopian neighborhood? You'd be correct in assuming that Fremont is home to some of the most progressive folks in Seattle.

By night it attracts a younger, rowdy college-age crowd, by day it's full of beatniks sipping coffee in the many coffee shops.

Fremont is home to Uneeda Burger, Homegrown, PCC, Flying Apron, Blue Moon Burgers, Revel and did I mention the Troll?

Three "no-wheat" symbols or less means limited gluten-free options, however they still do a great job catering to gluten-free.

NEIGHBORHOOD GUIDE

AGRODOLCE 🌾🌾🌾🌾

ⓘ *Italian*
  Not Dedicated Gluten-Free

📍 **Address:**
  709 N 35th St
  Seattle, WA 98103

📞 **(206) 547-9707**

🔗 www.agrodolcerestaurant.net

See full review on page 131.

BLUE MOON BURGERS 🌾🌾🌾🌾

ⓘ *Burger Joint*
  Not Dedicated Gluten-Free

📍 **Address:**
  703 N 34th St
  Seattle, WA 98103

📞 **(206) 547-1907**

🔗 www.bluemoonburgers.com

See full review on page 114.

EL CAMINO 🌾🌾🌾🌾

ⓘ *Mexican, Dinner & Weekend Brunch*
  Not Dedicated Gluten-Free

📍 **Address:**
  607 N 35th St
  Seattle, WA 98103

📞 **(206) 632-7303**

🔗 www.elcaminorestaurant.com

See full review on page 110.

NEIGHBORHOOD GUIDE

FLYING APRON 🌱🌱🌱🌱🌱

ⓘ *Gluten-Free Bakery*
    Dedicated Facility

📍 **Address:**
    3510 Fremont Ave N
    Seattle, WA 98103

📞 **(206) 442-1115**

🔗 www.flyingapron.com

See full review on page 102.

HOMEGROWN 🌱🌱🌱🌱

ⓘ *Sandwich and Soup Shop*
    Not Dedicated Gluten-Free

📍 **Address:**
    3416 Fremont Ave N
    Seattle, WA 98103

📞 **(206) 453-5232**

🔗 www.eathomegrown.com

See full review on page 21 and 148.

HUNGER 🌱🌱🌱🌱

ⓘ *Spanish, Dinner and Weekend Brunch*
    Not Dedicated Gluten-Free

📍 **Address:**
    3601 Fremont Ave N
    Seattle, WA 98103

📞 **(206) 402-4854**

🔗 www.hungerseattle.com

See full review on page 153.

NEIGHBORHOOD GUIDE

KAOSAMAI THAI RESTAURANT

ⓘ   *Thai*
Not Dedicated Gluten-Free

📍   **Address:**
404 N 36th St
Seattle, WA 98103

📞   **(206) 925-9979**

🔗   www.kaosamai.com

See full review on page 157.

PCC NATURAL MARKETS

ⓘ   *Natural and Organic Grocery Store*
Not Dedicated Gluten-Free

📍   **Address:**
600 N 34th St
Seattle, WA 98103

📞   **(206) 632-6811**

🔗   www.pccnaturalmarkets.com

See full review on page 127.

PIE

ⓘ   *Savory and Sweet Pies, Dessert*
Not Dedicated Gluten-Free

📍   **Address:**
3525 Fremont Ave
Seattle, WA 98103

📞   **(206) 436-8590**

🔗   www.sweetandsavorypie.com

See full review on page 95.

NEIGHBORHOOD GUIDE

REVEL 🌾🌾🌾🌾

ⓘ *Korean Fusion*
Not Dedicated Gluten-Free

📍 **Address:**
403 N 36th St
Seattle, WA 98103

📞 **(206) 547-2040**

🔗 www.revelseattle.com

See full review on page 112.

SILENCE-HEART NEST 🌾🌾🌾

ⓘ *Vegetarian, Breakfast and Lunch*
Not Dedicated Gluten-Free

📍 **Address:**
3508 Fremont Pl N
Seattle, WA 98103

📞 **(206) 633-5169**

🔗 www.silenceheartnest.com

See full review on page 161.

UNEEDA BURGER 🌾🌾🌾🌾

ⓘ *Burger Joint*
Not Dedicated Gluten-Free

📍 **Address:**
4306 Fremont Ave N
Seattle, WA 98103

📞 **(206) 547-2600**

🔗 www.uneedaburger.com

See full review on page 114.

NEIGHBORHOOD GUIDE

Green Lake

Green Lake is one of Seattle's many treasures. It's a lake, right in the middle of a beautiful neighborhood. Ducks, birds, squirrels and sometimes rabbits hop around this lake and so do local residents, especially when it's sunny.

It's a favorite for dog walkers, roller bladers and runners. On a sunny day, Green Lake looks like a fantastical, lush slice of heaven. If you are a regular, you are probably familiar with the dancing roller skater lady and the Spanish man offering language lessons.

Green Lake has a few gluten-free options as well. Green Lake Bar and Grill, Thrive (Roosevelt), Jodee's Desserts, Eva Restaurant and Garlic Jim's (Ravenna) are some of the few in this area.

Three "no-wheat" symbols or less means limited gluten-free options, however they still do a great job catering to gluten-free.

BENGAL TIGER 🌾🌾🌾🌾

ⓘ *Indian*
Not Dedicated Gluten-Free

📍 **Address:**
6509 Roosevelt Way NE
Seattle, WA 98115

📞 **(206) 985-0041**

🔗 www.bengaltigerwa.com

See full review on page 130.

NEIGHBORHOOD GUIDE

BOL PHO BISTRO 🌾🌾🌾🌾

ⓘ *Vietnamese*
   Not Dedicated Gluten-Free

📍 **Address:**
   918 NE 64th St
   Seattle, WA 98115

📞 **(206) 397-4782**

🔗 www.bolbistro.com

See full review on page 164.

EVA RESTAURANT 🌾🌾

ⓘ *American New*
   Not Dedicated Gluten-Free

📍 **Address:**
   2227 N 56th St
   Seattle, WA 98103

📞 **(206) 633-3538**

🔗 www.evarestaurant.com

See full review on page 98.

GARLIC JIM'S FAMOUS GOURMET PIZZA 🌾🌾🌾

ⓘ *Pizza Delivery*
   Not Dedicated Gluten-Free

📍 **Address:**
   2400 NE 65th St
   Seattle, WA 98115

📞 **(206) 524-5467**

🔗 www.garlicjims.com

See full review on page 142.

NEIGHBORHOOD GUIDE

JODEE'S DESSERTS

(i) *Raw Desserts*
Dedicated Facility

⦿ **Address:**
7214 Woodlawn Avenue NE
Seattle, WA 98115

☎ **(206) 525-2900**

🔗 www.jodeesdesserts.com

See full review on page 13 and 103.

GREENLAKE BAR AND GRILL

(i) *Bar and Grill*
Not Dedicated Gluten-Free

⦿ **Address:**
7200 East Green Lake Dr N
Seattle, WA 98115

☎ **(206) 729-6179**

🔗 www.neighborhoodgrills.com

See full review on page 94.

THRIVE

(i) *Raw, Vegan and Gluten-Free*
Dedicated Gluten-free Facility

⦿ **Address:**
1026 NE 65th St
Seattle, WA 98115

☎ **(206) 525-0300**

🔗 www.generationthrive.com

See full review on page 25 and 162.

NEIGHBORHOOD GUIDE

Greenwood

Greenwood is a cool little spot that struggles in food options, but really shines for nightlife. It's an affordable part of town and home to one of Seattle's first gluten-free merchants, RAZZiS Pizzeria.

Come to this area for a cider, pizza and a flamboyant art gallery show.

Three "no-wheat" symbols or less means limited gluten-free options, however they still do a great job catering to gluten-free.

RAZZiS PIZZA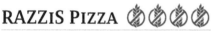

ⓘ   *Pizza Parlor*
     Not Dedicated Gluten-Free

◉   **Address:**
     8523 Greenwood Ave N
     Seattle, WA 98103

☎   **(206) 782-9005**

🔗   www.razzispizza.com

See full review on page 145.

STUMBLING GOAT BISTRO

ⓘ   *American New*
     Not Dedicated Gluten-Free

◉   **Address:**
     6722 Greenwood Ave N
     Seattle, WA 98103

☎   **(206) 784-3535**

🔗   www.stumblinggoatbistro.com

See full review on page 99.

Madison Park

If you are looking for the wealthy part of Seattle, you will find it in Madison Park. This neighborhood, still manages to be on the sweeter side blessing visitors with astounding beauty during the summer time. It sits aside Lake Washington, offering a few beaches for afternoon sun bathing.

Of the mercantile residents, Madison Park has a few boutiques and shops, as well as a handful of restaurants.

Three "no-wheat" symbols or less means limited gluten-free options, however they still do a great job catering to gluten-free.

CACTUS RESTAURANTS

ⓘ *Southwestern and Mexican Cuisine*
Not Dedicated Gluten-Free

📍 **Address:**
4220 E. Madison St
Seattle, WA 98112

📞 **(206) 324-4140**

🔗 www.cactusrestaurants.com

See full review on page 138.

CAFE FLORA

ⓘ *Vegetarian*
Not Dedicated Gluten-Free

📍 **Address:**
2901 E Madison St
Seattle, WA 98112

📞 **(206) 325-9100**

🔗 www.cafeflora.com

See full review on page 159.

NEIGHBORHOOD GUIDE

ESSENTIAL BAKING COMPANY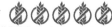

ⓘ   *Breakfast and Lunch Cafe*
    Not Dedicated Gluten-Free

📍   **Address:**
    2719 E Madison Street
    Seattle, WA 98112

📞   **(206) 328-0078**

🔗   www.essentialbaking.com

See full review on page 148.

Maple Leaf

One of the proudest up and coming neighborhoods in the city not known for nightlife but instead for cute, residential "Maple Leaf 4 Lifers" aka new families and craftsman houses. If you enjoy house gazing, Maple Leaf is a pleasurable little day walk. Make your way to the Maple Leaf Reservoir Park or to the handful of restaurants scattered along Roosevelt.

Maple Leaf is home to Roosevelt Alehouse, COA, Café Piccolo, Blue Saucer Cafe, Cloud City Coffee and Mojito.

Three "no-wheat" symbols or less means limited gluten-free options, however they still do a great job catering to gluten-free.

NEIGHBORHOOD GUIDE

BLUE SAUCER CAFE

(i) *Coffee Shop*
Not Dedicated Gluten-Free

Address:
9127 Roosevelt Way NE
Seattle, WA 98115

(206) 453-4955

www.bluesaucer.com

See full review on page 115.

CAFÉ PICCOLO

(i) *Italian*
Not Dedicated Gluten-Free

Address:
9400 Roosevelt Way NE
Seattle, WA 98115

(206) 957-1333

www.piccoloseattle.com

See full review on page 19 and 132.

COA

(i) *Mexican*
Not Dedicated Gluten-Free

Address:
7919 Roosevelt Way NE
Seattle, WA 98115

(206) 522-6179

www.coainseattle.com

See full review on page 139.

NEIGHBORHOOD GUIDE

MOJITO

ⓘ *Cuban Fusion*
   Not Dedicated Gluten-Free

📍 **Address:**
   7545 Lake City Way NE
   Seattle, WA 98115

📞 **(206) 525-3162**

🔗 www.mojito1.com

See full review on page 119.

ROOSEVELT ALEHOUSE

ⓘ *Bar and Grill*
   Not Dedicated Gluten-Free

📍 **Address:**
   8824 Roosevelt Way NE
   Seattle, WA 98115

📞 **(206) 527-5480**

🔗 www.rooseveltalehouse.com

See full review on page 95.

SNAPPY DRAGON

ⓘ *Chinese*
   Not Dedicated Gluten-Free

📍 **Address:**
   8917 Roosevelt Way NE
   Seattle, WA 98115

📞 **(206) 528-5575**

🔗 www.snappydragon.com

See full review on page 118.

NEIGHBORHOOD GUIDE

Queen Anne

Queen Anne is a somewhat regal neighborhood, sitting atop Seattle with stoic observation. The houses in this area are some of the oldest and largest in Seattle proper. Many have a more colonial look and are said to be haunted.

When I grew up on Queen Anne, it wasn't as trendy, but now it's a hive of activity. Lower on the hill you will find the younger crowd living in brick apartments, further up, you will find young families and retirees resting easy in their century-old homes.

Three "no-wheat" symbols or less means limited gluten-free options, however they still do a great job catering to gluten-free.

CEDERBERG TEA HOUSE 🌾🌾🌾

ⓘ *South African*
Not Dedicated Gluten-Free

📍 **Address:**
1417 Queen Anne Ave N
Seattle, WA 98109

📞 **(206) 285-1352**

🔗 www.cederbergteahouse.com

See full review on page 116.

I ❤ MY GFF 🌾🌾🌾🌾

ⓘ *Rice Bowls*
Dedicated Gluten-Free
Food Truck

Visit Website for Location:

🔗 www.ilovemygff.com

See full review on page 111.

MOD PIZZA 🌾🌾🌾

ⓘ *Pizza*
  Not Dedicated Gluten-Free

📍 **Address:**
  Seattle Center/Armory Building
  305 Harrison St
  Seattle, WA 98109

📞 **(206) 428-6315**

🔗 www.modpizza.com

See full review on page 143.

NEW YORK PIZZA & BAR 🌾🌾🌾🌾

ⓘ *Pizza Parlor*
  Not Dedicated Gluten-Free

📍 **Address:**
  500 Mercer St
  Seattle, WA 98109

📞 **(206) 913-2565**

🔗 www.newyorkpizzaandbar.com

See full review on page 144.

TEN MERCER 🌾🌾🌾

ⓘ *American New*
  Not Dedicated Gluten-Free

📍 **Address:**
  10 Mercer St
  Seattle, WA 98119

📞 **(206) 691-3723**

🔗 www.tenmercer.com

See full review on page 99.

NEIGHBORHOOD GUIDE

THE 5 SPOT 🌾🌾🌾

ⓘ *Breakfast and Brunch*
   Not Dedicated Gluten-Free

📍 **Address:**
   1502 Queen Anne Ave N
   Seattle, WA 98109

📞 **(206) 285-7768**

🔗 www.chowfoods.com

See full review on page 96.

TRADER JOE'S 🌾🌾🌾

ⓘ *Natural Grocery Store*
   Not Dedicated Gluten-Free

📍 **Address:**
   112 West Galer St
   Seattle, WA 98119

📞 **(206) 378-5536**

🔗 www.traderjoes.com

See full review on page 128.

WHOLE FOODS MARKETS 🌾🌾🌾🌾🌾

ⓘ *Natural Grocery Store*
   Not Dedicated Gluten-Free

📍 **Address:**
   2001 15th Ave W
   Seattle, WA 98119

📞 **(206) 352-5440**

🔗 www.wholefoodsmarket.com

See full review on page 129.

NEIGHBORHOOD GUIDE

ZAW 🌾🌾

ⓘ *Artisan Pizza*
   Not Dedicated Gluten-Free

📍 **Address:**
   1635 Queen Anne Ave N
   Seattle, WA 98109

📞 **(206) 787-1198**

🔗 www.zaw.com

See full review on page 146.

South Lake Union

It's called the new "Bellevue" of downtown, because South Lake Union is pretty much brand new and as chic as Seattle gets. Also known as the SLU, it's home to Seattle's techiest of folks and most of them work on Amazon's campus (also in SLU).

It's a nice part of town by day, but fairly sleepy by night. We suggest you venture up the hill (to Capitol Hill) if you are looking for more nightlife.

You won't go hungry in this neighborhood. Apparently, techies are pretty in touch with their food allergies too, because the SLU has more options for gluten-free than any other neighborhood.

South Lake Union is home to Nollie's Cafe, Cactus, Portage Bay Cafe, Yellow Dot Cafe, a plethora of Amazon cafes that carry Tarte Nouveau, Cuoco, Whole Foods and ZAW.

It's worth mentioning that during lunch hours Monday through Friday, you will find some 10-20 food trucks (with long lines) set up around this neighborhood, I ♥ My GFF and Contigo are among the frenzy.

NEIGHBORHOOD GUIDE

BLUE MOON BURGERS

ⓘ *Burger Joint*
Not Dedicated Gluten-Free

📍 **Address:**
920 Republican St
Seattle, WA 98109

📞 **(206) 652-0400**

🔗 www.bluemoonburgers.com

See full review on page 114.

CACTUS RESTAURANTS

ⓘ *Southwestern and Mexican Cuisine*
Not Dedicated Gluten-Free

📍 **Address:**
350 Terry Ave N
Seattle, WA 98109

📞 **206-913-2250**

🔗 www.cactusrestaurants.com

See full review on page 138.

CONTIGO

ⓘ *Modern Mexican*
Not Dedicated Gluten-Free
Food Truck

Visit website for daily locations.

🔗 www.contigoseattle.com

See full review on page 138.

CUOCO

ⓘ *Northern Italian*
Not Dedicated Gluten-Free

📍 **Address:**
310 Terry Ave N
Seattle, WA 98109

📞 **(206) 971-0710**

🔗 www.cuoco-seattle.com

See full review on page 132.

I ❤ MY GFF

ⓘ *Rice Bowls*
Dedicated Gluten-Free
Food Truck

Visit Website for Location.

🔗 www.ilovemygff.com

See full review on page 111.

NOLLIE'S CAFÉ

ⓘ *Sandwiches and Baked Goods*
Not Dedicated Gluten-Free

📍 **Address:**
1165 Harrison St
Seattle, WA 98109

📞 **(206) 402-6724**

🔗 www.nolliescafe.com

See full review on page 116.

NEIGHBORHOOD GUIDE

PORTAGE BAY CAFE

ⓘ *Breakfast and Lunch Cafe*
Not Dedicated Gluten-Free

📍 **Address:**
391 Terry Ave N
Seattle, WA 98109

📞 **(206) 462-6400**

🔗 www.portagebaycafe.com

See full review on page 23 and 111.

SEASTAR RESTAURANT AND RAW BAR

ⓘ *Seafood*
Not Dedicated Gluten-Free

📍 **Address:**
2121 Terry Ave #108
Seattle, WA 98109

📞 **(206) 462-4364**

🔗 www.seastarrestaurant.com

See full review on page 152.

WHOLE FOODS MARKETS

ⓘ *Natural Grocery Store*
Not Dedicated Gluten-Free

📍 **Address:**
2210 Westlake Ave
Seattle, WA 98121

📞 **(206) 621-9700**

🔗 www.wholefoodsmarket.com

See full review on page 129.

NEIGHBORHOOD GUIDE

YELLOW DOT CAFÉ 🌾🌾🌾

ⓘ *Sandwich Shop*
   Not Dedicated Gluten-Free

📍 **Address:**
   301 Westlake Ave N
   Seattle, WA 98109

📞 **(206) 381-9200**

🔗 www.yellowdotcafe.com

See full review on page 152.

ZAW 🌾🌾🌾

ⓘ *Artisan Pizza*
   Not Dedicated Gluten-Free

📍 **Address:**
   434 Yale Ave N
   Seattle, WA 98109

📞 **(206) 623-0299**

🔗 www.zaw.com

See full review on page 146.

University

You can tell from the name that the University area is home to mostly students from University of Washington. It's also home to a plethora of ethnic food, vegan cafés and other delicious fare.

The "Ave" as it's known, is scroungy, unmaintained and frequents quite a few loiterers. Don't judge this area by its cover, the surrounding merchants offer good service and food for the most part. If you trek down to University Village, you will see the polar opposite. This area has a lot of money, corporate chains and a nice, new outdoor mall. Both areas have gluten-free options, but you will find healthier options closer to the college.

Three "no-wheat" symbols or less means limited gluten-free options, however they still do a great job catering to gluten-free.

50 NORTH 🌾🌾🌾🌾

ⓘ *American New*
Not Dedicated Gluten-Free

📍 **Address:**
5001 25th Ave NE
Seattle, WA 98105

📞 **(206) 397-3939**

🔗 www.50northrestaurant.com

See full review on page 97.

CHACO CANYON CAFÉ 🌾🌾🌾🌾

ⓘ *Raw and Vegan Café*
Not Dedicated Gluten-Free

📍 **Address:**
4757 12th Ave NE
Seattle, WA 98105

📞 **(206) 522-6966**

🔗 www.chacocanyoncafe.com

See full review on page 147.

ESSENTIAL BAKING COMPANY

(i) *Breakfast and Lunch Cafe*
Not Dedicated Gluten-Free

📍 **Address:**
1604 N 34th Street
Seattle, WA 98103

📞 **(206) 545-0444**

🔗 www.essentialbaking.com

See full review on page 148.

FRAN'S CHOCOLATES

(i) *Chocolatier*
Dedicated Gluten-Free

📍 **Address:**
2626 NE University Village St
Seattle, WA 98105

📞 **(206) 528-9969**

🔗 www.franschocolates.com

See full review on page 147.

MAMMA MELINA
RISTORANTE & PIZZERIA

(i) *Italian*
Not Dedicated Gluten-Free

📍 **Address:**
5101 25th Ave NE
Seattle, WA 98105

📞 **(206) 632-2271**

🔗 www.mammamelina.com

See full review on page 133.

NEIGHBORHOOD GUIDE

MOD Pizza 🌾🌾🌾

ⓘ *Pizza*
Not Dedicated Gluten-Free

📍 **Address:**
1414 42nd St NE
Seattle, WA 98105

📞 **(206) 632-7111**

🔗 www.modpizza.com

See full review on page 143.

PCC Natural Markets 🌾🌾🌾🌾🌾

ⓘ *Natural and Organic Grocery Store*
Not Dedicated Gluten-Free

📍 **Address:**
6514 40th Ave NE
Seattle, WA 98115

📞 **(206) 526-7661**

🔗 www.pccnaturalmarkets.com

See full review on page 127.

Piatti Italian Restaurant 🌾

ⓘ *Italian*
Not Dedicated Gluten-Free

📍 **Address:**
University Village
2695 NE Village Lane
Seattle, WA 98105

📞 **(206) 524-9088**

🔗 www.piatti.com

See full review on page 133.

PORTAGE BAY CAFE 🌾🌾🌾🌾🌾

ⓘ *Breakfast and Lunch Cafe*
   Not Dedicated Gluten-Free

📍 **Address:**
   4130 Roosevelt Way NE
   Seattle, WA 98105

📞 **(206) 547-8230**

🔗 www.portagebaycafe.com

See full review on page 23 and 111.

RAM RESTAURANT & BREWERY 🌾🌾🌾

ⓘ *Bar & Grill*
   Not Dedicated Gluten-Free

📍 **Address:**
   2650 NE University Village St
   Seattle, WA 98105

📞 **(206) 525-3565**

🔗 www.theram.com

See full review on page 107.

TRADER JOE'S 🌾🌾🌾

ⓘ *Natural Grocery Store*
   Not Dedicated Gluten-Free

📍 **Address:**
   4555 Roosevelt Way NE
   Seattle, WA 98105

📞 **(206) 547-6299**

🔗 www.traderjoes.com

See full review on page 128.

NEIGHBORHOOD GUIDE

WAYWARD VEGAN CAFÉ 🌾🌾🌾🌾

(i)   *Vegan Café*
      Not Dedicated Gluten-Free

📍   **Address:**
     5253 University Way NE
     Seattle, WA 98105

📞   **(206) 524-0204**

🔗   www.waywardvegancafe.com

See full review on page 163.

Wallingford

Wallingford gives me the warm, fuzzies. In Danish it's called "hyggelig," (pronounced hoo-goo-lee) that special something that makes you feel at home. This area has a fairly chill, small shop and restaurant feel. It is the epitome of small businesses, which is my favorite kind of vibe.

You will find all kinds of ethnic food in this area like Thai, Sushi, Malaysian, Afghan and of course, Mexican.

Three "no-wheat" symbols or less means limited gluten-free options, however they still do a great job catering to gluten-free.

NEIGHBORHOOD GUIDE

MAY THAI 🌾🌾🌾🌾

ⓘ *Thai*
Not Dedicated Gluten-Free

📍 **Address:**
1612 N 45th St
Seattle, WA 98103

📞 **(206) 675-0037**

🔗 www.maythaiseattle.com

See full review on page 158.

KABUL 🌾🌾

ⓘ *Afghan, Mediterranean*
Not Dedicated Gluten-Free

📍 **Address:**
2301 N 45th St
Seattle, WA 98103

📞 **(206) 545-9000**

🔗 www.kabulrestaurant.com

See full review on page 137.

SATAY 🌾🌾

ⓘ *Malaysian Street Food*
Not Dedicated Gluten-Free

📍 **Address:**
1711 N 45th St
Seattle, WA 98103

📞 **(206) 547-0597**

🔗 www.satayseattle.com

See full review on page 136.

NEIGHBORHOOD GUIDE

SUTRA

(i) *Vegetarian, Vegan*
Not Dedicated Gluten-Free

📍 **Address:**
1605 N 45th St
Seattle, WA 98103

📞 **(206) 547-1348**

🔗 www.sutraseattle.com

See full review on page 161.

TNT TAQUERIA

(i) *Mexican, Tacos*
Not Dedicated Gluten-Free

📍 **Address:**
2114 N 45th St
Seattle, WA 98103

📞 **(206) 322-0124**

🔗 www.chowfoods.com/tnt-taqueria

See full review on page 141.

TROPHY CUPCAKES

(i) *Cupcakes and Desserts*
Not Dedicated Gluten-Free

📍 **Address:**
1815 N 45th St #209
Seattle, WA 98103

📞 **(206) 632-7020**

🔗 www.trophycupcakes.com

See full review on page 17 and 125.

NEIGHBORHOOD GUIDE

TEAHOUSE KUAN YIN 🌿🌿🌿

ⓘ *Tea*
   Not Dedicated Gluten-Free

📍 **Address:**
   1911 N 45th St
   Seattle, WA 98103

📞 **(206) 632-2055**

🔗 www.teahousekuanyin.com

See full review on page 157.

VEGAN CAKES BY JENNYMAC 🌿🌿🌿

ⓘ *Desserts*
   Not Dedicated Gluten-Free

📍 **Address:**
   4230 2nd Ave NE
   Seattle, WA 98105

📞 **(206) 495-2149**

🔗 www.vegancakesbyjennymac.com

See full review on page 163.

ZAW 🌿🌿🌿

ⓘ *Artisan Pizza*
   Not Dedicated Gluten-Free

📍 **Address:**
   4612 Stone Way
   Seattle, WA 98103

📞 **(206) 297-1334**

🔗 www.zaw.com

See full review on page 146.

NEIGHBORHOOD GUIDE

West Seattle

In the way west, more like South of downtown Seattle there exists a happy little island with happy little houses. Many folk vetured out to West Seattle to buy a modest house with a less inflated price tag near the beach. The only bummer is the West Seattle Bridge, which is one of the only direct routes there, has a bit of traffic during commuting hours.

You will find a handful of gluten-free restaurants like Catus, Matador, and Chaco Canyon Café. My guess is more options will pop in in the next year or two.

Three "no-wheat" symbols or less means limited gluten-free options, however they still do a great job catering to gluten-free

CACTUS RESTAURANTS

(i) *Southwestern and Mexican Cuisine*
Not Dedicated Gluten-Free

📍 **Address:**
2820 Alki Ave SW
Seattle, WA 98116

📞 **(206) 933-6000**

🔗 www.cactusrestaurants.com

See full review on page 138.

good happy hour menu.

free easy parking behind restaurant

CHACO CANYON CAFÉ

ⓘ *Raw and Vegan Café*
Not Dedicated Gluten-Free

📍 **Address:**
3770 SW Alaska St
Seattle, WA 98126

📞 **(206) 937-8732**

🔗 www.chacocanyoncafe.com

See full review on page 159.

MATADOR

ⓘ *Tex-Mex*
Not Dedicated Gluten-Free

📍 **Address:**
4546 California Ave. SW
Seattle, WA 98116

📞 **(206) 932-9988**

🔗 www.matadorseattle.com

See full review on page 140.

PCC NATURAL MARKETS

ⓘ *Natural and Organic Grocery Store*
Not Dedicated Gluten-Free

📍 **Address:**
2749 California Ave SW
Seattle, WA 98116

📞 **(206) 937-8481**

🔗 www.pccnaturalmarkets.com

See full review on page 127.

NEIGHBORHOOD GUIDE

TRADER JOE'S 🌾🌾🌾

ⓘ *Natural Grocery Store*
Not Dedicated Gluten-Free

📍 **Address:**
4545 Fauntleroy Way SW
Seattle, WA 98116

📞 **(206) 913-0013**

🔗 www.traderjoes.com

See full review on page 128.

ZAW 🌾🌾🌾

ⓘ *Artisan Pizza*
Not Dedicated Gluten-Free

📍 **Address:**
4151 Fauntleroy Way SW
Seattle, WA

📞 **(206) 859-5199**

🔗 www.zaw.com

See full review on page 146.

NEIGHBORHOOD GUIDE

PART 4: CUISINE GUIDE

American Diner

BISCUIT BITCH 🌾🌾🌾

(i) *Comfort Food, Breakfast, Lunch, Late Night*
   Not Dedicated Gluten-Free

📍 **Address:**
   1909 1st Ave
   Seattle, WA 98101

📞 **(206) 441-7999**

🔗 www.biscuitbitch.com

The name makes you wonder if Jesse Pinkman's character
from Breaking Bad opened his own restaurant after his
infamous meth-making career. Alas, he did not, but I still love
the name. Biscuit Bitch serves southern-inspired fixin's and
the city's best locally roasted coffee to Pike Place (the most
touristy place in the city). This is one of those diners on your
itinerary that should be visited right before nap hour. Soaked
in gravy, cheese, bacon and jalapenos, their biscuits are some
of the best gut-bombs in Seattle. Did we mention they have
gluten-free biscuits?

CAPITOL CIDER

(i) *Gluten-Free Pub*
Dedicated Gluten-Free

📍 **Address:**
818 E Pike St
Seattle, WA 98122

📞 **(206) 397-3564**

🔗 www.seattleciderbar.com

It's rare when a restaurant keeps their kitchen free of gluten, but Capitol Cider has done just that. I think this has earned them a place amongst the few who've gone above and beyond in the name of gluten allergies. They offer a unique menu of gluten-free gnocchi, chicken, fries, salads, steak frites and other upscale pub cuisine along with an array of ciders, cocktails, wine and beers (which do contain gluten).

CANYONS RESTAURANT

(i) *American*
Not Dedicated Gluten-Free

📍 **Address:**
15740 Redmond Way
Redmond, WA 98052

📞 **(425) 556-1390**

🔗 www.canyonsrestaurant.com

Canyons Restaurant is fairly accommodating, they have specially marked all items on their menu that can be made gluten-free and vegetarian. Redmond is not a place you will find yourself unless you happen to be wine tasting in Woodinville (it's neighbor) or visiting Microsoft, but it's good to know there are a few good options out east.

CHEESECAKE FACTORY

ⓘ *American*
  Not Dedicated Gluten-Free

◉ **Address:**
  700 Pike St
  Seattle, WA 98109

  Tacoma Mall

☎ **(206) 652-5400**

🔗 www.thecheesecakefactory.com

It's corporate and ALWAYS packed. I wouldn't brave it, but if you decide to, the Cheesecake Factory has a whole menu of gluten-free dishes, including a chocolate, gluten-free cheesecake.

EASTLAKE BAR AND GRILL

ⓘ *Bar and Grill*
  Not Dedicated Gluten-Free

◉ **Address:**
  2947 Eastlake Ave E
  Seattle, WA 98102

☎ **(206) 957-7777**

🔗 www.neighborhoodgrills.com

Under the I-5 bridge you will find the quaint little area of Eastlake. If you are in the neighborhood and craving a burger and fries, then Eastlake Bar and Grill is your spot. They carry gluten-free buns and pastas. Be sure to check with your server for other gluten-free options.

CUISINE GUIDE

GREENLAKE BAR AND GRILL

   (i)   *Bar and Grill*
       Not Dedicated Gluten-Free

   📍   **Address:**
       7200 East Green Lake Dr N
       Seattle, WA 98115

   📞   **(206) 729-6179**

   🔗   www.neighborhoodgrills.com

Greenlake Bar and Grill sits on the parameter of Green Lake. During the summer, it's the perfect spot for people watching and a burger. All gluten-free items and options are marked on their menu, but be sure to check with your server if something is not featured.

ICON GRILL 🌾🌾🌾

   (i)   *American*
       Not Dedicated Gluten-Free

   📍   **Address:**
       1933 5th Ave
       Seattle, WA 98101

   📞   **(206) 441-6330**

   🔗   www.icongrill.com

Icon Grill is one of those classic American restaurants with dark wood and place settings that make you feel small. They carry Maninis Gluten-free pasta and have marked every gluten-free dish on their menu for gluten-free diners. The food is decent and served in large portions, which might be why I feel like a wee little one there.

PIE 🌱🌱🌱

ⓘ *Savory and Sweet Pies, Dessert*
Not Dedicated Gluten-Free

📍 **Queen Anne/**
Seattle Center:
305 Harrison St
Seattle, WA 98109

📞 **(206) 428-6312**

📍 **Fremont:**
3525 Fremont Ave
Seattle, WA 98103

📞 **(206) 436-8590**

🔗 www.sweetandsavorypie.com

Pie, pie, me oh my. Pie is known for making just about every pie possible to man and guess what? They make gluten-free pies as well! Each day Pie makes one gluten-free flavor, both savory and sweet. Today, it could be the gluten-free Broccoli Cheddar and Strawberry Rhubarb, tomorrow Gluten-Free Creamy Kale with Apple and Gluten-Free Mango Blueberry. There is a $5.50 charge for gluten-free flavors and if you'd like to special order or have Pie cater your event, you can choose from over a hundred flavors on their website. Pie also serves Full Tilt ice cream.

ROOSEVELT ALEHOUSE 🌱🌱🌱🌱

ⓘ *Bar and Grill*
Not Dedicated Gluten-Free

📍 **Address:**
8824 Roosevelt Way NE
Seattle, WA 98115

📞 **(206) 527-5480**

🔗 www.rooseveltalehouse.com

Coined the "Railhouse," Roosevelt Alehouse is an above average pub food and a well-known Wednesday trivia night. Roosevelt Alehouse serves gluten-free pizza, sandwiches, burgers, quesadillas and chicken fingers. This pub also carries

Omission beer, which is a new (fantastic) gluten-free beer. They are a step above most bar food, everything is well-prepared with fresh ingredients.

THE 5 SPOT

ⓘ *Breakfast and Brunch*
Not Dedicated Gluten-Free

◉ **Address:**
1502 Queen Anne Ave N
Seattle, WA 98109

☎ **(206) 285-7768**

🔗 www.chowfoods.com

Themes are the name of the game at The 5 Spot. Their seasonal dishes are built around cities in the US, which decorate the walls in art, in food and if you are lucky in an audio tour tape playing in the restroom. Last time I was in, I listened to an audio tour of Alcatraz (a tribute to San Francisco), in the ladies' loo. In oddball-style, they will substitute toast and sandwich bread for the gluten-free variety, all you have to do is ask.

THE HI-LIFE

ⓘ *American*
Not Dedicated Gluten-Free

◉ **Address:**
5425 Russell Ave NW
Seattle, WA 98107

☎ **(206) 784-7272**

🔗 www.chowfoods.com/hi-life

Owned by Chow Foods, a chain of unique diners, the Hi-Life has gluten-free bread to substitute in sandwiches, toast and burgers. The food is typical American and super tasty. They serve breakfast, lunch and dinner.

CUISINE GUIDE

American New

50 NORTH 🌾🌾🌾🌾

ⓘ *American New*
   Not Dedicated Gluten-Free

📍 **Address:**
   5001 25th Ave NE
   Seattle, WA 98105

📞 **(206) 397-3939**

🔗 www.50northrestaurant.com

You will see on 50 North's menu that most items are available gluten-free and no they didn't just take out the gluten. They prepare alternative, gluten-free dishes like fish and chips, breaded and all. They also have fluffy gluten-free buns and desserts. During happy hour, their Waygu beef burger is only $5. Shhh, it's a secret.

BOKA RESTAURANT & BAR 🌾🌾🌾

ⓘ *American New/Northwest*
   Not Dedicated Gluten-Free

📍 **Address:**
   1010 First Ave
   Seattle, WA 98104

📞 **(206) 357-9000**

🔗 www.bokaseattle.com

If you are looking for a place that captures Northwest cuisine, BOKA is it. The restaurant serves breakfast, lunch and dinner and is also open late night. All dishes that can be made gluten-free are marked on their menu, many of which hail from the Northwest, like Taylor Shellfish. They have a moderate

CUISINE GUIDE

amount of gluten-free options, so you won't go hungry from salad-starvation.

EVA RESTAURANT 🌾🌾

ⓘ *American New*
Not Dedicated Gluten-Free

📍 **Address:**
2227 N 56th St
Seattle, WA 98103

📞 **(206) 633-3538**

🔗 www.evarestaurant.com

Eva is a delicious and healthy American New restaurant in the Green Lake/Tangletown area. Eva has multiple dishes that are gluten-free, like steak, fish, and chicken. All you have to do is ask, they will make a dish gluten-free if they can.

RAVISH 🌾

ⓘ *American New*
Not Dedicated Gluten-Free

📍 **Address:**
2956 Eastlake Ave E
Seattle, WA 98102

📞 **(206) 913-2497**

🔗 www.ravishoneastlake.com

Most of Ravish's choice menu items are swimming or baked in gluten, however there are a few healthier items like the Harissa Quinoa dish. I'd say eat here (despite how great their reviews are) for salad if you are gluten-free.

STUMBLING GOAT BISTRO

(i)   *American New*
     Not Dedicated Gluten-Free

📍   **Address:**
     6722 Greenwood Ave N
     Seattle, WA 98103

📞   **(206) 784-3535**

🔗   www.stumblinggoatbistro.com

I just love Stumbling Goat, it's quaint and always delivers an
excellent meal. It's expensive, but a fantastic, upscale place
to enjoy finer dining. The servers are as friendly as can be
(probably because they are older and wiser citizens) and more
than happy to make any dish gluten-free if they are able.

TEN MERCER

(i)   *American New*
     Not Dedicated Gluten-Free

📍   **Address:**
     10 Mercer St
     Seattle, WA 98119

📞   **(206) 691-3723**

🔗   www.tenmercer.com

Ten Mercer has dedicated an entire menu to gluten-free
items. You have a choice of seafood, poultry, beef, risotto
dishes and the like. When I was there last they over salted my
fish to the point where it tasted like it had been marinated
in baking soda. They did remake the dish and it was much
better, but my experience has been hit or miss for taste.

CUISINE GUIDE

TERRA PLATA

ⓘ *Modern American*
Not Dedicated Gluten-Free

📍 **Address:**
1501 Melrose Ave
Seattle, WA 98122

📞 **(206) 325-1501**

🔗 www.terraplata.com

I love it when a restaurant commits their brand to organic, locally-sourced food. Terra Plata has a delicious take on Modern American cuisine, they will also accomodate guests with gluten allergies, just ask your server.

Bakeries

COFFEE & A SPECIALTY BAKERY

ⓘ *Café and Bakery*
Dedicated Gluten-Free

📍 **Address:**
1500 Western Ave
Seattle, WA 98101

📞 **(206) 280-7946**

If you are exploring Pike Place and happen to make it one street down towards the waterfront (Western), which you can do through one of the elevators, you will find a hidden little gem called Coffee & A Specialty Bakery. The owner (a trained pastry chef) isn't gluten-free, but certainly likes a challenge, so she decided to make gluten-free baked goods that were actually delicious and she succeeded. Visit earlier in the day for the best array of pastries, both savory and sweet.

CUPCAKE ROYALE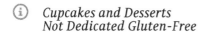

ⓘ *Cupcakes and Desserts*
Not Dedicated Gluten-Free

📍 **Ballard:**
2052 NW Market St
Seattle, WA 98107

📞 **(206) 883-7656**

📍 **Capitol Hill:**
1111 East Pike St
Seattle, WA 98122

📞 **(206) 883-7656**

📍 **Bellevue:**
21 Bellevue Way NE
Bellevue, WA 98004

📞 **(206) 883-7656**

📍 **Downtown:**
108 Pine St
Seattle, WA 98101

📞 **(206) 883-7656**

📍 **Madrona:**
1101 34th Ave
Seattle, WA 98122

📞 **(206) 883-7656**

📍 **West Seattle:**
4556 California Ave SW
Seattle, WA 98116

📞 **(206) 883-7656**

📍 **Queen Anne:**
1935 Queen Anne Ave
Seattle, WA 98109

📞 **(206) 883-7656**

🔗 www.cupcakeroyale.com

You name the (obscure) holiday and Cupcake Royale will have a special cupcake to fit the day. To better serve their gluten-free customers they also offer one flavor of gluten-free cupcake, double fudge brownie with a frosting of your choice. It is a decent cupcake, if you happen to be in one of their locations and need a quick sugar fix.

CUISINE GUIDE

EDEN B BAKERY 🌾🌾🌾🌾

(i) *Bakery and Café*
Dedicated Gluten-Free

📍 **Address:**
120 116th Ave NE
Bellevue, WA 98004

📞 **(425) 462-2224**

🔗 www.edenbbakery.com

Eden B Bakery is located in a car dealership, so the location is a little different, but they serve and bake up some of the most outstanding 100% gluten-free goods. You will find cupcakes, muffins, ding dongs, macaroons and cookies. They also have breakfast, lunch pizzas and sandwiches.

FLYING APRON 🌾🌾🌾🌾🌾

(i) *Gluten-Free Bakery*
Dedicated Facility

📍 **Fremont:**
3510 Fremont Ave N
Seattle, WA 98103

📞 **(206) 442-1115**

📍 **Redmond:**
16541 Redmond Way, #E
Redmond, WA 98052

📞 **(206) 442-1115**

🔗 www.flyingapron.com

Flying Apron is actually a very appropriate name. Their vast and varied menu has some of the best gluten-free baked goods in Seattle, both savory and sweet. Everything in this bakery is gluten-free. They have improved 100% since their first little shop opened in the University District. You can also find their baked goods at all PCC locations.

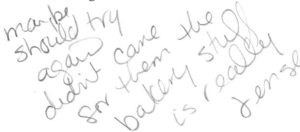

maybe should try again didn't care the for them bakery stuff is really dense

GUILT FREE GOODNESS 🌾🌾🌾🌾

ⓘ *Bakery*
   Dedicated Gluten-Free

📍 **Address:**
   219 Broadway E
   Seattle, WA 98102

📞 **(360) 794-5266**

🔗 www.guilt-free-goodness.com

I can't say they are entirely "guilt-free," sugar is sugar and carbs are carbs. Guilt Free Goodness specializes in gluten-free breads, cookies, mixes, muffins and pizza crusts to name a few. This bakery/café primarily uses rice flours and is located in the upper floor of the building.

JODEE'S DESSERTS 🌾🌾🌾🌾🌾

ⓘ *Raw Desserts*
   Dedicated Facility

📍 **Address:**
   7214 Woodlawn Avenue NE
   Seattle, WA 98115

📞 **(206) 525-2900**

🔗 www.jodeesdesserts.com

And the Gods gave us Jodee's. Each little pie is a slice of heaven, made with only coconut, agave, and love. Everything is gluten-free (they do use oat crusts, which some gluten-free folks react to), vegan, and made with low-glycemic sweeteners. These little desserts are expensive, one slice is $7.00, but worth every bite. See my write up on Jodee's Desserts in our Best-of section.

SWEET CAKES BAKERY 🌾🌾🌾🌾

(i) *Bakery and Desserts*
Dedicated Facility

📍 **Address:**
128 Park Lane
Kirkland, WA 98033

📞 **(425) 821-6565**

🔗 www.sweetcakeskirkland.com

How sweet it is to be loved by Sweet Cakes Bakery. This sweet little bakery makes gluten-free birthday, special-occasion, and wedding cakes as well as cupcakes. We have not sampled them, but have heard from our followers they are quite delicious.

TROPHY CUPCAKES 🌾🌾🌾🌾

(i) *Cupcakes and Desserts*
Not Dedicated Gluten-Free

📍 **Bellevue:**
700 110th Ave NE
Bellevue, WA 98004

📞 **(425) 361-0033**

📍 **Downtown:**
Pacific Place
Third Floor, 600 Pine St
Seattle, WA 98101

📞 **(206) 632-7020**

📍 **Wallingford:**
1815 45th St
Seattle, WA 98103

📞 **(206) 632-7020**

📍 **University:**
2612 NE Village Lane
Seattle, WA 98105

📞 **(206) 632-7020**

🔗 www.trophycupcakes.com

The blue and white stripes are Trophy's sugary calling card; you can find them at 4 locations around town. These cupcake experts just started carrying 9 gluten-free cupcakes – red velvet, triple chocolate, salted caramel, Neapolitan, chocolate-vanilla, samoa, chocolate-espresso-bean, snowball and chocolate peanut butter. Watch your waistline! Eek!

Bar and Grill

CAPITOL CIDER

(i) *Gluten-Free Pub*
     Dedicated Gluten-Free

📍 **Address:**
    818 E Pike St
    Seattle, WA 98122

📞 **(206) 397-3564**

🔗 www.seattleciderbar.com

It's rare when a restaurant keeps their kitchen free of gluten, but Capitol Cider has done just that. I think this has earned them a place amongst the few who've gone above and beyond in the name of gluten allergies. They offer a unique menu of gluten-free gnocchi, chicken, fries, salads, steak frites and other upscale pub cuisine along with an array of ciders, cocktails, wine and beers (which do contain gluten).

EASTLAKE BAR AND GRILL

(i) *Bar and Grill*
     Not Dedicated Gluten-Free

📍 **Address:**
    2947 Eastlake Ave E
    Seattle, WA 98102

📞 **(206) 957-7777**

🔗 www.neighborhoodgrills.com/eastlake

Under the I-5 bridge you will find the quaint little area of Eastlake. If you are in the neighborhood and craving a burger and fries, then Eastlake Bar and Grill is your spot. They carry gluten-free buns and pastas. Be sure to check with your server for other gluten-free options.

ICON GRILL 🔥🔥🔥

ⓘ   *American*
   Not Dedicated Gluten-Free

📍 **Address:**
   1933 5th Ave
   Seattle, WA 98101

📞 **(206) 441-6330**

🔗 www.icongrill.com

Icon Grill is one of those classic American restaurants with dark wood and place settings that make you feel small. They carry Maninis Gluten-free pasta and have marked every gluten-free dish on their menu for gluten-free diners. The food is decent and served in large portions, which might be why I feel like a wee little one there.

GREENLAKE BAR AND GRILL 🔥🔥🔥

ⓘ   *Bar and Grill*
   Not Dedicated Gluten-Free

📍 **Address:**
   7200 East Green Lake Dr N
   Seattle, WA 98115

📞 **(206) 729-6179**

🔗 www.neighborhoodgrills.com/greenlake

Greenlake Bar and Grill sits on the parameter of Green Lake. During the summer, it's the perfect spot for people watching and a burger. All gluten-free items and options are marked on their menu, but be sure to check with your server if something is not featured.

CUISINE GUIDE

RAM RESTAURANT & BREWERY

(i) *Bar & Grill*
     Not Dedicated Gluten-Free

📍 **University:**   📍 **Northgate:**
    2650 NE University   401 NE Northgate Way,
    Village St   Ste 1102
    Seattle, WA 98105   Seattle, WA 98125

📞 **(206) 525-3565**   📞 **(206) 364-8000**

🔗 www.theram.com

If you are looking for a sausage feast of dudes and lots of
TV's playing various sports channels, then stop in RAM.
The corporate chain serves typical bar food, but somehow
managed to put together a stellar (separate) gluten-free
menu. They didn't just take out the gluten either, they use
gluten-free breads and went as far as making their own rice
flour tortilla with the same texture and taste as a regular
flour tortilla. ✓this out in Tacoma

ROOSEVELT ALEHOUSE

(i) *Bar and Grill*
     Not Dedicated Gluten-Free

📍 **Address:**
    8824 Roosevelt Way NE
    Seattle, WA 98115

📞 **(206) 527-5480**

🔗 www.rooseveltalehouse.com

Coined the "Ralehouse," Roosevelt Alehouse is an above
average pub food and a well-known Wednesday trivia night.
Roosevelt Alehouse serves gluten-free pizza, sandwiches,
burgers, quesadillas and chicken fingers. This pub also carries
Omission beer, which is a new (fantastic) gluten-free beer.
They are a step above most bar food, everything is well-
prepared with fresh ingredients.

CUISINE GUIDE

Bed and Breakfast

AUNT LOUISE'S SECRET 🌾🌾🌾🌾🌾

ⓘ *Bed and Breakfast*
   Not Dedicated Gluten-Free

📍 **Address:**
   16004 NE 203rd PL
   Woodinville, WA 98072

📞 **(206) 351-8858**

🔗 www.auntlouisessecret.com

Aunt Louise's Secret is a quaint bed and breakfast located in Woodinville, WA that caters to just about any type of guest. I am mentioning them here because they will prepare gluten-free meals for their guests if it is mentioned during booking. The innkeeper also caters to the wine tasting tourist, providing transportation to and from wineries and concerts.

MERITAGE MEADOWS INN 🌾🌾🌾🌾🌾

ⓘ *Bed and Breakfast*
   Not Dedicated Gluten-Free

📍 **Address:**
   21407 NE Union Hill Rd
   Redmond, WA 98053

📞 **(425) 487-4019**

🔗 www.meritagemeadows.com

This is a beautiful lodge nestled out in the backwoods of Redmond, WA. The estate sits on a large property, undisturbed by neighbors or car traffic. The innkeepers make their own wine, cook guests food from scratch, and offer fun workshops and classes to participate in. When you book, request gluten-free meals, they will make sure all of your food is gluten-free. If you care to venture off the property, Marymoor Park is nearby for a beautiful stroll or the Burke-Gilman trail offers a splendid day biking adventure. The inn is near downtown Redmond, so if it gets a little too quiet, there is a nice outdoor mall and shopping area just 10 minutes away.

Breakfast and Lunch

BISCUIT BITCH 🌾🌾🌾

ⓘ   *Comfort Food, Breakfast, Lunch, Late Night*
    Not Dedicated Gluten-Free

📍   **Address:**
    1909 1st Ave
    Seattle, WA 98101

📞   **(206)-441-7999**

🔗   www.biscuitbitch.com

The name makes you wonder if Jesse Pinkman's character from Breaking Bad opened his own restaurant after his infamous meth-making career. Alas, he did not, but we still love the name. Biscuit Bitch serves southern-inspired fixin's and the city's best locally roasted coffee to Pike Place (the most touristy place in the city). This is one of those diners on your itinerary that should be visited right before nap hour. Soaked in gravy, cheese, bacon and jalapenos, these biscuits are some of the best gut-bombs in Seattle. Did we mention they have gluten-free biscuits?

CUISINE GUIDE

EL CAMINO ✺✺✺✺

ⓘ *Mexican, Dinner & Weekend Brunch*
Not Dedicated Gluten-Free

📍 **Address:**
607 N 35th St
Seattle, WA 98103

📞 **(206) 632-7303**

🔗 www.elcaminorestaurant.com

El Camino (the restaurant) is actually a whole lot cooler
than the car. It's Mexican, but more Oaxacan-style with
a Northwest twist. Many dishes are naturally gluten-free
because the preferred tortilla is made in-house from corn.
Weekend brunch is a delicious menu of huevos, chorizo,
chilaquiles and more. Don't miss it! El Camino stopped
serving brunch for awhile and had so many requests to bring
it back, it's here again who knows for how long.

HOMEGROWN ✺✺✺✺

ⓘ *Sandwich and Soup Shop*
Not Dedicated Gluten-Free

📍 **Capitol Hill:**
1531 Melrose Ave
Seattle, WA 98122

📞 **(206)-682-0935**

📍 **Downtown:**
2nd Ave and Marion St
Seattle, WA

📞 **(206) 624-1329**

📍 **Fremont:**
3416 Fremont Ave N
Seattle, WA 98103

📞 **(206) 453-5232**

📍 **Queen Anne:**
2201 Queen Anne Ave N
Seattle, WA 98119

📞 **(206) 217-4745**

🔗 www.eathomegrown.com

Homegrown serves deliciously thick gluten-free sandwiches,
soups, and salads at all three locations. In Seattle-style,

everything is organic and locally grown. When I was in the Fremont location they had run out of soup by early afternoon, so get there early, especially if it's a cold day. Serves both breakfast and lunch sandwiches. See my write up on Homegrown in our Best-of section.

I ♥ My GFF 🌾🌾🌾🌾🌾

ⓘ *Rice Bowls*
Dedicated Gluten-Free
Food Truck

Visit Website for Location.

🔗 www.ilovemygff.com

I ♥ My GFF! It's a pretty bare bones food truck, but doesn't fall short of delivering flavorful healthy gluten-free lunch food. They specialize in rice and quinoa bowls with meats, veggies and other sauces. Check their website for daily location.

Portage Bay Cafe 🌾🌾🌾🌾🌾

ⓘ *Breakfast and Lunch Cafe*
Not Dedicated Gluten-Free    *awesome food amazing fills you up!*

📍 **Ballard:**
2821 NW Market St
Seattle, WA 98107

📍 **University:**
4130 Roosevelt Way NE
Seattle, WA 98105

📞 (206) 783-1547

📞 (206) 547-8230

📍 **South Lake Union:**
391 Terry Ave N
Seattle, WA 98109

📞 (206) 462-6400

🔗 www.portagebaycafe.com

This is one of Seattle's favorites. Portage Bay Cafe serves

all organic and hormone-free dishes. All three locations serve homemade gluten-free cuisine for breakfast and lunch, which include sandwiches, pancakes and a thick, mesmerizing French toast. Be sure to visit the toppings bar to add a mountain of berries, fruit, and whip to any sweet breakfast option. See my write up on Portage Bay Cafe in our Best-of section.

REVEL

(i) *Korean Fusion*
Not Dedicated Gluten-Free

📍 **Address:**
403 N 36th St
Seattle, WA 98103

📞 **(206) 547-2040**

🔗 www.revelseattle.com

Revel is a rustic yet chic, Korean fusion restaurant in Fremont with many gluten-free options. My favorite dishes are the pancake with pork and short rib rice bowl with egg yolk. Be sure to let your server know you are gluten-free. Revel serves breakfast, lunch and dinner.

THE HI-LIFE

(i) *American*
Not Dedicated Gluten-Free

📍 **Address:**
5425 Russell Ave NW
Seattle, WA 98107

📞 **(206) 784-7272**

🔗 www.chowfoods.com

Owned by Chow Foods, a chain of unique diners, the Hi-Life has gluten-free bread to substitute in sandwiches, toast and burgers. The food is typical American, but super tasty. They serve breakfast, lunch and dinner.

Burger Joints

8 oz Burger Bar 🌾🌾🌾

(i) *Burger Joint*
     Not Dedicated Gluten-Free

📍 **Address:**
    1401 Broadway
    Seattle, WA 98122

📞 **(206) 466-5989**

🔗 www.8ozburgerbarsea.com

If you like a mean, tall burger that you can hardly fit in your mouth, then 8 oz Burger Bar is where you should go stat. They carry a gluten-free bun so all of us allergics can enjoy the pleasantries of dislocating our jaws in the name of greasy beef burger eating.

BLUE MOON BURGERS 🌾🌾🌾🌾

ⓘ *Burger Joint*
Not Dedicated Gluten-Free

📍 **Capitol Hill:**
523 Broadway East
Seattle, WA 98102

📞 **(206) 325-2000**

📍 **South Lake Union:**
920 Republican St
Seattle, WA 98109

📞 **(206) 652-0400**

📍 **Fremont:**
703 N 34th St
Seattle, WA 98138

📞 **(206) 547-1907**

🔗 www.bluemoonburgers.com

I'm 'over the moon' for Blue Moon Burgers when I want a to-go classic burger. Blue Moon uses free-range meat and a lot of grease, so I'm not complaining. They serve beef, salmon, and chicken gluten-free burgers as well as gluten-free chicken fingers, tater tots, sandwiches and sauces.

UNEEDA BURGER 🌾🌾🌾🌾

ⓘ *Burger Joint*
Not Dedicated Gluten-Free

📍 **Address:**
4306 Fremont Ave N
Seattle, WA 98103

📞 **(206) 547-2600**

🔗 www.uneedaburger.com

You really do need a gluten-free burger from this place. They use Olivia Superfree buns and offer a variety of interesting burgers that require lots of napkins! Don't leave without enjoying one of their signature milkshakes.

Cafés

BLUE SAUCER CAFE 🌀

(i) *Coffee Shop*
Not Dedicated Gluten-Free

📍 **Address:**
9127 Roosevelt Way NE
Seattle, WA 98115

📞 **(206) 453-4955**

🔗 www.bluesaucer.com

Blue Saucer Cafe is a sweet little coffee shop on the corner of Roosevelt and 92nd who serves gluten-free desserts only. They carry the most delicious cakes, which are delivered Tuesday and Thursday. They sell out quick so you might miss them. They also carry gluten-free brownies, cookies and whoopie pies.

COFFEE & A SPECIALTY BAKERY 🌀🌀🌀🌀🌀

(i) *Café and Bakery*
Dedicated Gluten-Free

📍 **Address:**
1500 Western Ave
Seattle, WA 98101

📞 **(206) 280-7946**

If you are exploring Pike Place and happen to make it one street down towards the waterfront (Western), which you can do through one of the elevators, you will find a hidden little gem called Coffee & A Specialty Bakery. The owner (a trained pastry chef) isn't gluten-free, but certainly likes a challenge, so she decided to make gluten-free baked goods that were actually delicious and she succeeded. Visit earlier in the day for the best array of pastries, both savory and sweet.

CEDERBERG TEA HOUSE

(i) *South African*
     Not Dedicated Gluten-Free

📍 **Address:**
    1417 Queen Anne Ave N
    Seattle, WA 98109

📞 **(206) 285-1352**

🔗 www.cederbergteahouse.com

Cederberg is a very unique, new tea house and café. The owners are from South Africa, so all of their baked goods are of the South African variety and most are not gluten-free. That said, they do carry gluten-free bread for their delicious sandwiches. My favorite is the bacon and banana sandwich.

NOLLIE'S CAFÉ

(i) *Sandwiches and Baked Goods*
     Not Dedicated Gluten-Free

📍 **Address:**
    1165 Harrison St
    Seattle, WA 98109

    (206) 402-6724

🔗 www.nolliescafe.com

Nollie's Café is a hole-in-the-wall sandwich shop that will make any sandwich with gluten-free bread. They also have several gluten-free homemade treats as well. I really enjoyed eating here when I worked for Amazon, it was never busy and the staff was super friendly.

CUISINE GUIDE

YELLOW DOT CAFÉ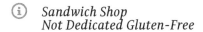

ⓘ *Sandwich Shop*
   Not Dedicated Gluten-Free

📍 **Address:**
   301 Westlake Ave N
   Seattle, WA 98109

📞 **(206) 381-9200**

🔗 www.yellowdotcafe.com

Yellow Dot is a busy little café that will serve any sandwich on gluten-free bread. They do not have a dedicated grill for warm sandwiches, but if you are not celiac it's a good to-go option.

Chinese

PF CHANG'S

ⓘ *Chinese*
   Not Dedicated Gluten-Free

📍 **Bellevue:**
   Bellevue Square
   525 Bellevue Square
   Bellevue, WA 98004

📞 **(425) 637-3582**

📍 **Downtown:**
   Westlake Center
   400 Pine St #136
   Seattle, WA 98101

📞 **(206) 393-0070**

📍 **Lynnwood:**
   Alderwood Mall
   3000 184th St SW #912
   Lynnwood, WA 98037

📞 **(425) 921-2100**

🔗 www.pfchangs.com

CUISINE GUIDE

PF Chang's is one of those big, corporate, international Chinese restaurant chains that happens to offer a gluten-free menu. Who knew? I consider them a socially responsible business for doing so. The food is a few cuts above other Chinese restaurants and they are very careful (almost paranoid) you are not glutenized.

SNAPPY DRAGON

ⓘ   *Chinese*
    Not Dedicated Gluten-Free

📍   **Address:**
    8917 Roosevelt Way Northeast
    Seattle, WA 98115

📞   **(206) 528-5575**

🔗   www.snappydragon.com

Somehow Snappy Dragon has a cult following in Seattle, so much so, residents of the Eastside will venture into the city just to visit and I'm not sure why. I think the food is a little too normal for me, which may suggest I'm bananas. It could be true... They have an entire gluten-free menu on their website for download and available when you dine-in.

Cuban

MOJITO 🌾🌾🌾

ⓘ *Cuban Fusion*
Not Dedicated Gluten-Free

📍 **Address:**
7545 Lake City Way NE
Seattle, WA 98115

📞 **(206) 525-3162**

🔗 www.mojito1.com

They don't really know they are gluten-free, but Mojito's entire Cuban/S. American menu aside from the lunch sandwiches, are gluten-free. They serve large portions of slow-roasted pork, baked fish, plantain cakes, and much more! The staff is not afraid to dance with female patrons on a busy night, so have your dance shoes on before you go.

Desserts

FRAN'S CHOCOLATES 🌾🌾🌾🌾🌾

ⓘ *Chocolatier*
   Dedicated Gluten-Free

📍 **Bellevue:**
   10036 Main St
   Seattle, WA 98004

📞 **(425) 453-1698**

📍 **Downtown:**
   1325 1st Ave
   Seattle, WA 98101

📞 **(206) 682-0168**

📍 **University:**
   2626 NE University
   Village St
   Seattle, WA 98105

📞 **(206) 528-9969**

🔗 www.franschocolates.com

At first it was by accident, Fran's Chocolates was using a (wheat-based) glucose syrup in the making of their caramels and their supplier stopped producing it. Along with impetus from gluten-free customers, Fran's replaced their sweeteners with tapioca syrup, eliminated all gluten production in their kitchens, and now test all of their products for gluten just to be sure. So technically, Fran's is certified gluten-free (by the Food Allergy Research and Resource Program) showing less than 5 ppm (undetectable) levels of gluten. So now you have another reason to buy their smooth and delectable chocolates, you're welcome.

CUISINE GUIDE

FULL TILT ICE CREAM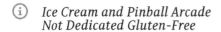

ⓘ *Ice Cream and Pinball Arcade*
Not Dedicated Gluten-Free

📍 **Ballard:**
5453 Leary Ave NW
Seattle, WA 98107

📞 **(206) 297-3000**

📍 **Columbia City:**
5041 Rainier Ave S
Seattle, WA 98118

📞 **(206) 226-2740**

📍 **University:**
4759 Brooklyn Ave NE
Seattle, WA 98105

📞 **(206) 524-4406**

📍 **White Center**
9629 16th Ave SW
Seattle, WA 98106

📞 **(206) 767-4811**

🔗 www.fulltilticecream.com

I feel like I revert back to my angst-ridden teen years when I hang out at Full Tilt. Pinball and arcade games were all the rage back then. Then the ice cream bangs out this superior flavor-fusion like Mayan Chocolate or cantalope with black pepper, and your like, "am I in some kind of perfect, euphoric nexus of tomfoolery?" They have more vegan ice creams than any other ice creamery and occassionally will have a gluten-free cookie dough ice cream by Skydottir Cookies.

CUPCAKE ROYALE 🌾🌾🌾

ⓘ *Cupcakes and Desserts*
Not Dedicated Gluten-Free

📍 **Ballard:**
2052 NW Market St
Seattle, WA 98107

📞 **(206) 883-7656**

📍 **Bellevue:**
21 Bellevue Way NE
Bellevue, WA 98004

📞 **(206) 883-7656**

📍 **Capitol Hill:**
1111 East Pike St
Seattle, WA 98122

📞 **(206) 883-7656**

📍 **Downtown:**
108 Pine St
Seattle, WA 98101

📞 **(206) 883-7656**

📍 **Madrona:**
1101 34th Ave
Seattle, WA 98122

📞 **(206) 883-7656**

📍 **Queen Anne:**
1935 Queen Anne Ave
Seattle, WA 98109

📞 **(206) 883-7656**

📍 **West Seattle:**
4556 California Ave SW
Seattle, WA 98116

📞 **(206) 883-7656**

🔗 www.cupcakeroyale.com

You name the (obscure) holiday and Cupcake Royale will have a special cupcake to fit the day. To better serve their gluten-free customers they also offer one flavor of gluten-free cupcake, double fudge brownie with a frosting of your choice. It is a decent cupcake, if you happen to be in one of their locations and need a quick sugar fix.

HOT CAKES MOLTEN CHOCOLATE ✿✿✿✿

ⓘ *Desserts*
   Not Dedicated Gluten-Free

📍 **Address:**
   5427 Ballard Ave NW
   Seattle, WA 98107

📞 **(206) 420-3431**

🔗 www.getyourhotcakes.com

They had me at hot and molten chocolate. Naturally gluten-free and worth writing home about, I can't give you enough reasons to visit for dessert. Be sure to ask your server to specify which desserts are gluten-free. They also serve shakes, cocktails and wine.

JODEE'S DESSERTS ✿✿✿✿✿

ⓘ *Raw Desserts*
   Dedicated Facility

📍 **Address:**
   7214 Woodlawn Avenue NE
   Seattle, WA 98115

📞 **(206) 525-2900**

🔗 www.jodeesdesserts.com

And the Gods gave us Jodee's. Each little pie is a slice of heaven, made with only coconut, agave, and love. Everything is gluten-free (they do use oat crusts, which some gluten-free folks react to), vegan, and low-glycemic sweeteners. These little desserts are expensive, one slice is $7.00, but worth every bite. See my write up on Jodee's Desserts in our Best-of section.

CUISINE GUIDE

MIRO TEA 🌱🌱🌱🌱🌱

ⓘ *Tea Shop, Crêperie, Desserts*
Not Dedicated Gluten-Free, but almost!

📍 **Address:**
5405 Ballard Ave NW
Seattle, WA 98107

📞 **(206) 782-6832**

🔗 www.mirotea.com

Miro Tea 'crêpes it real' in the most hipster-ish part of Ballard. Serving sweet and savory crêpes, this Tea Haus specializes in 100+ choices of herbal teas and has replaced almost all of their baked goods with gluten-free options for all the allergics out there. I recommend this Cêprerie for remote working and lunching options. See my write up on Miro Tea in our Best-of section.

PIE 🌱🌱🌱

ⓘ *Savory and Sweet Pies, Dessert*
Not Dedicated Gluten-Free

📍 **Queen Anne/**
Seattle Center:
305 Harrison St
Seattle, WA 98109

📞 **(206) 428-6312**

📍 **Fremont:**
3525 Fremont Ave
Seattle, WA 98103

📞 **(206) 436-8590**

🔗 www.sweetandsavorypie.com

Pie, pie, me oh my. Pie is known for making just about every pie possible to man and guess what? They make gluten-free pies as well! Each day Pie makes one gluten-free flavor, both savory and sweet. Today, it could be the gluten-free Broccoli Cheddar and Strawberry Rhubarb, tomorrow Gluten-Free Creamy Kale with Apple and Gluten-Free Mango Blueberry. There is a $5.50 charge for gluten-free flavors and if you'd like

to special order or have Pie cater your event, you can choose
from over a hundred flavors on their website. Pie also serves
Full Tilt ice cream.

SWEET CAKES BAKERY

ⓘ *Desserts*
Dedicated Facility

📍 **Address:**
128 Park Lane
Kirkland, WA 98033

📞 **(425) 821-6565**

🔗 www.sweetcakeskirkland.com

How sweet it is to be loved by Sweet Cakes Bakery. This
sweet little bakery makes gluten-free birthday, special-
occasion, and wedding cakes as well as cupcakes. We have not
sampled them, but have heard from our followers they are
quite delicious.

TROPHY CUPCAKES

ⓘ *Cupcakes and Desserts*
Not Dedicated Gluten-Free

📍 **Bellevue:**
700 110th Ave NE #260
Bellevue, WA 98004

📞 **(425) 361-0033**

📍 **Downtown:**
Pacific Place
Third Floor, 600 Pine St
Seattle, WA 98101

📞 **(206) 632-7020**

📍 **Wallingford:**
1815 45th St
Seattle, WA 98103

📞 **(206) 632-7020**

📍 **University:**
2612 NE Village Lane
Seattle, WA 98105

📞 **(206) 632-7020**

🔗 www.trophycupcakes.com

CUISINE GUIDE

The blue and white stripes are Trophy's sugary calling card; you can find them at 4 locations around town. These cupcake experts just started carrying 9 gluten-free cupcakes; red velvet, triple chocolate, salted caramel, Neapolitan, chocolate-vanilla, samoa, chocolate-espresso-bean, snowball and chocolate peanut butter. Watch your waistline! Eek!

VEGAN CAKES BY JENNYMAC 🌾🌾🌾

(i) *Desserts*
Not Dedicated Gluten-Free

📍 **Address:**
4230 2nd Ave NE
Seattle, WA 98105

📞 **(206) 495-2149**

🔗 www.vegancakesbyjennymac.com

I haven't actually ordered a cake or dessert from Jenny, but I see she does offer gluten-free options. She gets a five star rating and seems to be the place to go if you are allergic to multiple items like eggs, soy or sugar.

Grocery

JANELL'S GLUTEN-FREE MARKET 🌾🌾🌾🌾🌾

(i) *Grocery*
Dedicated Gluten-Free

📍 **Address:**
7024 Evergreen Way
Everett, WA 98203

📞 **(425) 347-3500**

🔗 www.janellsglutenfreemarket.com

If you are looking for one place that carries every gluten-free item known to man, you should stop into Janell's, which is far outside of any Seattle area I mention in this book. It's in a land called Everett, that whilst not be mentioned again. I only mention them because they are a grocery store free of gluten. Inside this mecca of gluten-free groceries you will find breads, baking mixes and flours, cookies, pasta, beers and ciders and take-n-bake pizzas. Need we go on?

PCC NATURAL MARKETS

(i) *Natural and Organic Grocery Store*
Not Dedicated Gluten-Free

Fremont:
600 N 34th St
Seattle, WA 98103

(206) 632-6811

Edmonds:
9803 Edmonds Way
Edmonds, WA 98020

(425) 275-9036

Issaquah:
1810 12th Ave NW
Issaquah, WA 98027

(425) 369-1222

Green Lake:
7504 Aurora Ave N
Seattle, WA 98103

(206) 525-3586

Kirkland:
10718 NE 68th
Kirkland, WA 98033

(425) 828-4622

Redmond:
11435 Avondale Rd NE
Redmond, WA 98052

(425) 285-1400

Seward Park:
5041 Wilson Ave S
Seattle, WA 98118

(206) 723-2720

University/Ravenna:
6514 40th Ave NE
Seattle, WA 98115

(206) 526-7661

West Seattle:
2749 California Ave SW
Seattle, WA 98116

(206) 937-8481

www.pccnaturalmarkets.com

CUISINE GUIDE

I remember when PCC was a tiny little co-op in Kirkland, stocked wall to wall with tofu, bulk food and hippies. PCC has come a long way from their tofu-loving days. The market is a marvel of gluten-free artisan pastries, as well as local and sustainable meats, dairy and veggies. You will still find a few hippies roaming around the supplement aisle, but now they have cell phones and are reveling in the organic wonderland of other delicious treats.

All 9 Seattle and Eastside locations carry Flying Apron, Olivia Superfree, Udi's, Rudi's and many other local and well-known gluten-free products. They've been stepping up their gluten-free deli options as well. Be sure to check out their deli section for pre-made gluten-free sandwiches and other to-go meal options.

brown rice tortillas—great but need to be heated 1st / gluten free bread & bagels! / cupcakes

TRADER JOE'S ❀❀❀

ⓘ *Natural Grocery Store*
Not Dedicated Gluten-Free

📍 **Ballard:**
4609 14th Ave NW
Seattle, WA 98107
📞 (206) 783-0498

📍 **Bellevue:**
15563 NE 24th St
Bellevue, WA 98007
📞 (425) 641-5069

📍 **Capitol Hill:**
1700 Madison St
Seattle, WA 98122
📞 (206) 322-7268

📍 **Kirkland:**
12632 120th Ave NE
Kirkland, WA 98034
📞 (425) 823-1685

📍 **Queen Anne:**
112 West Galer St
Seattle, WA 98119
📞 (206) 378-5536

📍 **Redmond:**
15932 Redmond Way
Redmond, WA 98052
📞 (425) 883-1624

📍 **University:**
4555 Roosevelt Way NE
Seattle, WA 98105
📞 (206) 547-6299

📍 **West Seattle:**
4545 Fauntleroy Way SW
Seattle, WA 98116
📞 (206) 913-0013

🔗 www.traderjoes.com

Trader Joe's is known for cheap, natural groceries but not as much for gluten-free. That said, they are starting to carry more gluten-free products like Udi's bread, cupcakes, cookies and crackers.

WHOLE FOODS MARKETS 🌾🌾🌾🌾🌾

(i) *Natural Grocery Store*
   Not Dedicated Gluten-Free

📍 **Bellevue:**
   888 116th Ave NE
   Bellevue, WA 98004

📞 **(425) 462-1400**

📍 **Redmond:**
   17991 Redmond Way
   Redmond, WA 98052

📞 **(425) 881-2600**

📍 **Green Lake/Ravenna:**
   1026 NE 64th St
   Seattle, WA 98155

📞 **(206) 985-1500**

📍 **South Lake Union:**
   2210 Westlake Ave
   Seattle, WA 98121

📞 **(206) 621-9700**

📍 **Queen Anne:**
   2001 15th Ave W
   Seattle, WA 98119

📞 **(206) 352-5440**

🔗 www.wholefoodsmarket.com

It's a little bit like heaven with a heavy price tag, despite the cost, Whole Foods does a stand-up job catering to the allergic. All Seattle and Eastside locations carry some of the best gluten-free brands on the market including Udi's, Rudi's, Essential Baking Company, Maninis, their own GF brand, and other local gluten-free products.

dairy free frosting

CUISINE GUIDE

Indian

ANNAPURNA CAFE

ⓘ *Indian/Tibetan*
Not Dedicated Gluten-Free

📍 **Address:**
1833 Broadway
Seattle, WA 98122

📞 **(206) 320-7770**

🔗 www.annapurnacafe.com

Annapurna is located in the basement of a building on
Broadway, so you have to know it's there. They serve Indian
and Tibetan food, so it's a little different than your run-of-
the-mill Indian restaurant. You won't be disappointed by the
quality of their food, which is served hot and full of exotic
flavors. Ask your server which items are gluten-free.

BENGAL TIGER

ⓘ *Indian*
Not Dedicated Gluten-Free

📍 **Address:**
6509 Roosevelt Way NE
Seattle, WA 98115

📞 **(206) 985-0041**

🔗 www.bengaltigerwa.com

You won't find a friendlier restaurateur than Chef Uddin.
He makes a point to greet guests personally if he is working.
There have been times where he made me a special lamb dish
not on the menu, just so I could try it, at no charge. Custom
lamb dishes are not a regular offering, so stick to the menu

and you will find Bengal Tiger to be one of the best Indian restaurants around with many naturally occurring gluten-free dishes. Chef Uddin tells me he is working on a gluten-free naan, which should be available soon.

Italian

AGRODOLCE ✎✎✎✎

(i) *Italian*
Not Dedicated Gluten-Free

📍 **Address:**
709 N 35th St
Seattle, WA 98103

📞 **(206) 547-9707**

🔗 www.agrodolcerestaurant.net

If you don't know Chef Maria Hines, you may have seen her on Iron Chef. She is quite the buzz name here in Seattle. Her new restaurant, Agrodolce, is a casual and welcoming trattoria featuring Italy's finest coastal cuisine. All dishes are expertly handmade with organic and sustainable ingredients from the Pacific Northwest. Not only is Agrodolce sustainable, they also serve gluten-free spaghetti and will make almost any dish gluten-free on request.

CAFÉ PICCOLO

(i) *Italian*
Not Dedicated Gluten-Free

📍 **Address:**
9400 Roosevelt Way Northeast
Seattle, WA 98115

📞 **(206) 957-1333**

🔗 www.piccoloseattle.com

Even though this little Italian restaurant is small and in a residential area, it's known for upscale Italian food. They also serve gluten-free lasagna, ravioli, spaghetti, fettuccine, meat dishes, and bread, skyrocketing themselves to be one of the best gluten-free Italian restaurants in Seattle. The food is gourmet and command gourmet prices, but it's worth every penny. See my write up on Café Piccolo in our Best-of section.

CUOCO

(i) *Northern Italian*
Not Dedicated Gluten-Free

📍 **Address:**
310 Terry Ave N
Seattle, WA 98109

📞 **(206) 971-0710**

🔗 www.cuoco-seattle.com

Cuoco is a Tom Douglas gourmet restaurant in South Lake Union. If you have heard his name and can't place the face, he's the big red-headed dude who wears crocs while he cooks. They have gluten-free dinner options listed on their website and use Maninis Gluten-free Pasta for their macaroni dish. They may sub out other items as well, but you will have to double check with them.

CUISINE GUIDE

MAMMA MELINA RISTORANTE & PIZZERIA

(i) *Italian*
Not Dedicated Gluten-Free

📍 **Address:**
5101 25th Ave NE
Seattle, WA 98105

📞 **(206) 632-2271**

🔗 www.mammamelina.com

"Mamma Mia" they have gluten-free! Mamma Melina's serves Maninis Gluten-free Pasta in their spaghetti and rigatoni dishes. You have to ask for them to do that and there is an extra surcharge.

PIATTI ITALIAN RESTAURANT

(i) *Italian*
Not Dedicated Gluten-Free

📍 **Address:**
University Village
2695 NE Village Lane
Seattle, WA 98105

📞 **(206) 524-9088**

🔗 www.piatti.com

Located in University Village, Piatti has a gluten-free menu that is fairly impressive. They also use Maninis Gluten-free bread and pasta for their paninis and pasta dishes.

CUISINE GUIDE

SAGE'S RESTAURANT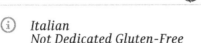

ⓘ   *Italian*
     Not Dedicated Gluten-Free

📍 **Address:**
     15916 NE 83rd Street
     Redmond, WA 98052

📞 **(425) 881-5004**

🔗 www.sagesrestaurant.com

Sage's created an entire gluten-free menu for diners to make it easier to dine gluten-free. That said they just removed all the wheat, pasta, and bread out of the dishes.

THE PINK DOOR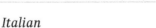

ⓘ   *Italian*
     Not Dedicated Gluten-Free

📍 **Address:**
     1919 Post Alley
     Seattle, Pike Place Market

📞 **(206)-443-3241**

🔗 www.thepinkdoor.net

Known for burlesque and quirky décor in Post Alley, The Pink Door, will make you a panini with gluten-free bread. Be sure to ask what other Italian options can be made gluten-free.

TULIO RISTORANTE 🌾🌾🌾

ⓘ *Italian*
Not Dedicated Gluten-Free

📍 **Address:**
1100 5th Ave
Seattle, WA 98101

📞 **(206) 624-5500**

🔗 www.tulio.com

Tulio is a great example of a restaurant who jumped on the bandwagon of gluten-free, but never delivered legit gluten-free options. Yes, some of their dishes can be made without gluten, but many cannot and are average at best in flavor. That said, if you are in the area, they are a 3 star option.

Korean

REVEL 🌾🌾🌾🌾

ⓘ *Korean Fusion*
Not Dedicated Gluten-Free

📍 **Address:**
403 N 36th St
Seattle, WA 98103

📞 **(206) 547-2040**

🔗 www.revelseattle.com

Revel is a rustic yet chic, Korean fusion restaurant in Fremont with many gluten-free options. My favorite dishes are the pancake with pork and short rib rice bowl with egg yolk. Be sure to let your server know you are gluten-free. Revel serves breakfast, lunch and dinner.

CUISINE GUIDE

Malaysian

SATAY 🌾🌾

ⓘ *Malaysian Street Food*
   Not Dedicated Gluten-Free

📍 **Address:**
   1711 N 45th St
   Seattle, WA 98103

📞 **(206) 547-0597**

🔗 www.satayseattle.com

Satay is a flavorful little spot with many naturally gluten-free options. Choose your meat and they will satay it up for you. All dishes are served with rice, salad, coconut milk, and chili pepper dressing. Ask your server if you suspect a dish might have gluten.

Mediterranean

ANDALUCA 🌾🌾🌾

ⓘ *Mediterranean*
   Not Dedicated Gluten-Free

📍 **Address:**
   407 Olive Way
   Seattle, WA 98101

📞 **(206)-382-6999**

🔗 www.andaluca.com

Andaluca is a higher-end Mediterranean restaurant serving breakfast and dinner in the Mayflower Hotel. While the price point may be a little higher, they cater to gluten allergies by serving an entire gluten-free menu.

KABUL 🌾🌾

(i) *Afghan, Mediterranean*
Not Dedicated Gluten-Free

📍 **Address:**
2301 N 45th St
Seattle, WA 98103

📞 **(206) 545-9000**

🔗 www.kabulrestaurant.com

Kabul's cuisine hails from the Afghan variety. Many of their dishes are naturally gluten-free and full of Mediterranean flavors like cardamom and garlic yogurt sauce. Please check with your server for gluten-free options.

MAMNOON 🌾🌾🌾

(i) *Middle Eastern, Mediterranean*
Not Dedicated Gluten-Free

📍 **Address:**
1508 Melrose Ave
Seattle, WA 98122

📞 **(206) 906-9606**

🔗 www.mamnoonrestaurant.com

Mamnoon is a super swanky Mediterranean restaurant across the street from Taylor Shellfish. It is one of the better (new) Mediterranean restaurants in Seattle in fact. They have gluten-free crackers to munch on while your dinner is prepared. My favorites are the chicken, beets and yogurt/cucumber side. Unfortunately, the lamb dishes have gluten, which are outstanding here. Be sure to check which dishes are gluten-free with your server.

CUISINE GUIDE

Mexican/Southwestern

CACTUS RESTAURANTS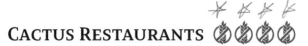

(i) *Southwestern and Mexican Cuisine*
   Not Dedicated Gluten-Free

📍 **Bellevue:**
535 Bellevue Way SE
Bellevue, WA 98004

📞 **(425) 455-4321**

📍 **Kirkland:**
121 Park Ln
Kirkland, WA 98033

📞 **(425) 893-9799**

📍 **Madison Park:**
4220 East Madison St
Seattle, WA 98112

📞 **(206) 324-4140**

📍 **South Lake Union:**
350 Terry Ave N
Seattle, WA 98109

📞 **(206) 913-2250**

📍 **West Seattle:**
2820 Alki Ave SW
Seattle, WA 98116

📞 **(206) 933-6000**

🔗 www.cactusrestaurants.com

Cactus is quite the hot spot for Southwest Mexican food in Seattle. On their menu they have marked which dishes can be made gluten-free, there are quite a few spicy and flavorful options.

CONTIGO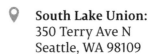

(i) *Modern Mexican*
   Not Dedicated Gluten-Free
   Food Truck

Visit website for daily locations.

🔗 www.contigoseattle.com

A posh little food truck with fiery modern Mexican food, Contigo will make many of their dishes gluten-free. Their location changes daily, please visit their website for locations.

COA 🌾🌾🌾

ⓘ *Mexican*
Not Dedicated Gluten-Free

📍 **Address:**
7919 Roosevelt Way NE
Seattle, WA 98115

📞 **(206) 522-6179**

🔗 www.coainseattle.com

Coa is the little Mexican restaurant that could. The restaurant occupies an old house on the corner of 80th and Roosevelt. Prior to its residency, the location had a few restaurants attempts by other business owners, but Coa is proving to be a hit with considerable staying power. It's a humble eatery that delivers an exceptional flavor and most items are naturally gluten-free (and marked on the menu). Stop in for happy hour and get juicy tacos for $2 each.

EL CAMINO 🌾🌾🌾🌾

ⓘ *Mexican, Happy Hour, Dinner & Late Night*
Not Dedicated Gluten-Free

📍 **Address:**
607 N 35th St
Seattle, WA 98103

📞 **(206) 632-7303**

🔗 www.elcaminorestaurant.com

El Camino is actually a whole lot cooler than the car. It's Mexican, but more Oaxacan-style with a Northwest twist. Many dishes are naturally gluten-free because the preferred

CUISINE GUIDE

tortilla is made in-house from corn. If you like mole sauce, cheese, carnitas and guacamole, visit during happy hour or dinner for a rich and spicy meal.

LITTLE WATER CANTINA 🌾🌾🌾

(i) *Mexican, Tacos*
Not Dedicated Gluten-Free

📍 **Address:**
2865 Eastlake Ave E
Seattle, WA 98102

📞 **(206) 397-4940**

🔗 www.littlewatercantina.com

In the summer, Little Water Cantina has a great view of Lake Union. On their busy patio, you can watch the boats glide by while munching on fresh guacamole and corn chips. For dinner, try the soft and juicy coca-cola and coconut milk marinated carnitas. Most items are naturally gluten-free, but clarify with your server first.

Tacoma too

MATADOR 🌾🌾🌾

(i) *Tex-Mex*
Not Dedicated Gluten-Free

📍 **Ballard:**
2221 NW Market St
Seattle, WA 98107

📞 **(206) 297-2855**

📍 **West Seattle:**
4546 California Ave. SW
Seattle, WA 98116

📞 **(206) 932-9988**

📍 **Redmond:**
7824 Leary Way NE
Redmond, WA 98052

📞 **(425) 883-2855**

Tacoma

🔗 www.matadorseattle.com

CUISINE GUIDE

It's kind of hip, dark and loud, but the food is pretty darn good. Matador has added a gluten-free menu, which is brimming with delicious gluten-free Tex-Mex options. My favorite thing on the menu has to be the nachos. Piled high and goopy with cheese - Matador knows how to make a nacho plate a gut-bomb. In fact, Matador probably has the best nachos in town, but don't just try the nachos, everything else is fantastic.

TNT TAQUERIA

(i) *Mexican, Tacos*
     Not Dedicated Gluten-Free

📍 **Address:**
     2114 N 45th St
     Seattle, WA 98103

📞 **(206) 322-0124**

🔗 www.chowfoods.com/tnt-taqueria

What TNT is most well-known for is delicious, juicy little tacos, served on soft (gf) corn tortillas. Your taco choices include al pastor, braised chicken, beef brisket, chorizo, carne asada, papas dulce & kale, hominy & spinach, and maximo. Did we mention they have breakfast too? If you are drooling now, put down this book and head straight there. They are open until 10 pm.

Pizza

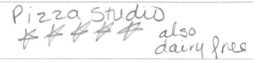

Pizza Studio
★ ★ ★ ★ also
dairy free

GARLIC JIM'S FAMOUS GOURMET PIZZA

(i) *Pizza Delivery*
Not Dedicated Gluten-Free

Bellevue:
10445 NE 4th St
Bellevue, WA 98004

(425) 455-5467

Bothell:
18404 120th Ave NE
Bothell, WA 98011

(425) 483-5555

Edmonds:
9796 Edmonds Way
Edmonds, WA 98020

(425) 771-5467

Kirkland:
9758 NE 119th Way
Kirkland, WA 98034

(425) 307-1122

Kirkland:
8431 122nd Ave NE
Kirkland, WA 98033

(425) 822-8881

Redmond:
11523 Avondale Rd NE
Redmond, WA 98052

(425) 861-9000

www.garlicjims.com

Who doesn't want a pipin' hot pizza delivered to their door? Garlic Jim's will make any flavor pizza on a gluten-free crust. Garlic Jim's is a pizza delivery or pick-up shop, they do not have dine-in seating.

MAMMA MELINA
RISTORANTE & PIZZERIA 🌾🌾

ⓘ *Italian*
   Not Dedicated Gluten-Free

📍 **Address:**
   5101 25th Ave NE
   Seattle, WA 98105

📞 **(206) 632-2271**

🔗 www.mammamelina.com

"Mamma Mia" they have gluten-free! Mamma Melina's will
sub out their spaghetti or rigatoni with Maninis Gluten-free
Pasta. You have to ask for them to do that and there is an
extra surcharge.

MOD PIZZA 🌾🌾 *Some are very slow & burn the crust*
Tacoma too

ⓘ *Pizza*
   Not Dedicated Gluten-Free

📍 **Bellevue:**
   317 Bellevue Way NE
   Bellevue, WA 98004

📞 **(425) 455-0141**

📍 **Downtown:**
   1302 6th Ave
   Seattle, WA 98101

📞 **(206) 332-0200**

📍 **Queen Anne/
   Seattle Center:**
   Armory Building
   305 Harrison St
   Seattle, WA 98109

📞 **(206) 428-6315**

🔗 www.modpizza.com

📍 **Redmond:**
   8900 161st Ave NE
   Redmond, WA 98052

📞 **(425) 497-5104**

📍 **University District:**
   1414 42nd St NE
   Seattle, WA 98105

📞 **(206) 632-7111**

*Tacoma Mall
Tacoma
Latewood
Towne Center*

*Pizza Studio
Latewood town center*

MOD Pizza is a fun pizza parlor that lets you mix and match flavors. They have a gluten-free crust, but don't recommend it for the ultra sensitive since it is created in an environment with other gluten products.

NEW YORK PIZZA & BAR

ⓘ *Pizza Parlor*
Not Dedicated Gluten-Free

📍 **Address:**
500 Mercer St
Seattle, WA 98109

📞 **(206) 913-2565**

🔗 www.newyorkpizzaandbar.com

New York Pizza & Bar serves an expansive a menu of gluten-free items. Worth a stop in if you are craving pizza in Queen Anne.

PALERMO RESTAURANT

ⓘ *Italian, Pizza*
Not Dedicated Gluten-Free

📍 **Ballard:**
2005 NW Market St
Seattle, WA 98107

📞 **(206) 297-2727**

📍 **Capitol Hill:**
350 15th Ave E
Seattle, WA 98112

📞 **(206)-322-3875**

🔗 www.palermopizzaseattle.com
🔗 www.palermorestaurant.com

It's a simple pizza and pasta joint, that delivers a solid gluten-free pizza. Their pasta is quite delicious as well. We have heard feedback from other readers that the quality can be hit or miss, so don't have too high of expectations.

RAZZiS PIZZA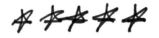

ⓘ *Pizza Parlor*
   Not Dedicated Gluten-Free

📍 **Address:**
   8523 Greenwood Ave N
   Seattle, WA 98103

📞 **(206) 782-9005**

🔗 www.razzispizza.com

100% love this place have a gluten free menu, gluten free vegan menu - gluten free vegan desserts & garlic Bread!

Formerly Romio's Pizza and the first to offer a HUGE gluten-free menu. RAZZiS have every gluten-free Italian dish you never knew you wanted including focaccia sandwiches, gyros, pizza, pasta, lasagna, ravioli, spaghetti, and desserts. It's an old-shool, nostalgic, Americanized Italian joint known for their comfort food. Don't eat too much, stomach-aches will ensue.

they have another location in Seattle

ROMIO'S PIZZA *(Counter service)*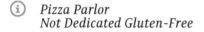

ⓘ *Pizza Parlor*
   Not Dedicated Gluten-Free

📍 **Bellevue:**   📍 **Kirkland:**
   3615 Factoria Blvd SE   11422 NE 124th St
   Bellevue, WA 98006   Kirkland, WA 98034

📞 **(425) 747-3000**   📞 **(425) 820-3300**

🔗 www.romiospizzafactoria.com

🔗 www.romioskirkland.com

Romio's is a franchise, so some of their locations carry gluten-free options and some don't. These particular locations carry gluten-free options. Their pizza is good, no complaints here.

CUISINE GUIDE

ZAW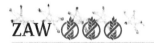

ⓘ *Artisan Pizza*
Not Dedicated Gluten-Free

📍 **Capitol Hill:**
1424 E. Pine St
Seattle, WA 98122

📞 **(206)-325-5528**

📍 **Kirkland:**
339 Kirkland Ave
Kirkland, WA 98033

📞 **(425) 298-4443**

📍 **South Lake Union:**
434 Yale Ave N
Seattle, WA 98109

📞 **(206) 623-0299**

📍 **Mercer Island:**
Tabit Village Square
7635 SE 27th St
Mercer Island, WA
98040

📞 **(206) 232-0515**

📍 **Redmond:**
8145 161st Ave NE
Redmond, WA 98052

📞 **(425) 952-4420**

📍 **Queen Anne:**
1635 Queen Anne Ave
Seattle, WA 98109

📞 **(206) 787-1198**

📍 **Wallingford:**
4612 Stone Way N
Seattle, WA 98103

📞 **(206) 297-1334**

📍 **Wedgewood:**
7320 35th Ave NE
Seattle, WA 98115

📞 **(206) 658-2929**

📍 **West Seattle:**
4151 Fauntleroy Way SW
Seattle, WA

📞 **(206) 859-5199**

🔗 www.zaw.com

Fresh ingredients plus creative pizza flavors equals
ZAW. It's an artisan pizza shop that will bake any of their
artisan flavors on a gluten-free crust. Everything here is
a little healthier than what you see at a typical pizza joint,
which suffers in grease points, but excels in keeping the
waistline trim.

CUISINE GUIDE

Sandwiches

CEDERBERG TEA HOUSE ⬮⬮⬮⬮

ⓘ *South African*
Not Dedicated Gluten-Free

📍 **Address:**
1417 Queen Anne Ave N
Seattle, WA 98109

📞 **(206) 285-1352**

🔗 www.cederbergteahouse.com

Cederberg is a very unique, new tea house and café. The owners are from South Africa, so all of their baked goods are of the South African variety and most are not gluten-free. That said, they do carry gluten-free bread for their delicious sandwiches. My favorite is the bacon and banana sandwich.

CHACO CANYON CAFÉ ⬮⬮⬮⬮

ⓘ *Raw and Vegan Café*
Not Dedicated Gluten-Free

📍 **University:**
4757 12th Ave NE
Seattle, WA 98105

📞 **(206) 522-6966**

📍 **West Seattle:**
3770 SW Alaska St
Seattle, WA 98126

📞 **(206) 937-8732**

🔗 www.chacocanyoncafe.com

For the vegan and raw enthusiast, Chaco Canyon Café serves up a menu of 90-97% organic sandwiches, salads, bowls and treats. Everything is vegan and some items are gluten-free.

CUISINE GUIDE

ESSENTIAL BAKING COMPANY 🌾🌾🌾🌾🌾

ⓘ *Breakfast and Lunch Cafe*
Not Dedicated Gluten-Free

📍 **Bellevue:**
990 102nd Avenue NE
Bellevue, WA 98004

📞 **(206) 876-3770**

📍 **Wallingford:**
1604 N 34th Street
Seattle, WA 98103

📞 **(206) 545-0444**

📍 **Madison:**
2719 E Madison Street
Seattle, WA 98112

📞 **(206) 328-0078**

📍 **Georgetown:**
5601 1st Avenue South
Seattle, WA 98108

📞 **(206) 876-3746**

🔗 www.essentialbaking.com

Essential Baking Company did a good thing. They came out with their own gluten-free sandwich breads and rolls. This bread maker/café is well-known in Seattle for being one of the best artisan bread makers. Now they have put themselves on the map as one of the best gluten-free bread makers as well. Oh and they will make you a sandwich on their bread at every café location, how do you like them bread rolls?

HEALEO 🌾🌾🌾🌾

ⓘ *Juice, Supplements, and Lunch*
Not Dedicated Gluten-Free

📍 **Address:**
1520 15th Ave
Seattle, WA 98122

📞 **(206)-453-5066**

🔗 www.healeo.com

Not only can you suck down a detoxifying beet, carrot, ginger juice at Healeo, but you can also get a gluten-free egg sandwich drenched in Pepper Jack cheese or a tempting gluten-free pizza. Healeo is mostly known for an array of supplements, smoothies, vegetable juices, and health shots, but hey I am happy to see they added in some substantial lunch menu items to munch on as well.

#106

550 - 106th Ave NE

HOMEGROWN

Bellevue WA 98004

877-567.9240

ⓘ *Sandwich and Soup Shop*
   Not Dedicated Gluten-Free

📍 **Capitol Hill:**
1531 Melrose Ave
Seattle, WA 98122

📞 **(206)-682-0935**

📍 **Fremont:**
3416 Fremont Ave N
Seattle, WA 98103

📞 **(206) 453-5232**

📍 **Downtown:**
2nd Ave and Marion St
Seattle, WA

📞 **(206) 624-1329**

📍 **Queen Anne:**
2201 Queen Anne Ave N
Seattle, WA 98119

📞 **(206) 217-4745**

🔗 www.eathomegrown.com

Redmond
Sammamish

Homegrown serves deliciously thick gluten-free sandwiches, soups, and salads at all three locations. In Seattle-style, everything is organic and locally grown. When I was in the Fremont location they had run out of soup by early afternoon, so get there early, especially if it's a cold day. Serves both breakfast and lunch sandwiches. See my write up on Homegrown in our Best-of section.

PORTAGE BAY CAFE

(i) *Breakfast and Lunch Cafe*
Not Dedicated Gluten-Free

📍 **Ballard:**
2821 NW Market St
Seattle, WA 98107

📞 **(206) 783-1547**

📍 **South Lake Union:**
391 Terry Ave N
Seattle, WA 98109

📞 **(206) 462-6400**

📍 **University:**
4130 Roosevelt Way NE
Seattle, WA 98105

📞 **(206) 547-8230**

🔗 www.portagebaycafe.com

This is one of Seattle's favorites. Portage Bay Cafe serves all organic and hormone-free dishes. All three locations serve homemade gluten-free cuisine for breakfast and lunch, which include sandwiches, pancakes and a thick, mesmerizing French toast. Be sure to visit the toppings bar to add a mountain of berries, fruit, and whip to any sweet breakfast option. See my write up on Portage Bay Cafe in our Best-of section.

RAZZiS PIZZA

(i) *Pizza Parlor*
Not Dedicated Gluten-Free

📍 **Address:**
8523 Greenwood Ave N
Seattle, WA 98103

📞 **(206) 782-9005**

🔗 www.razzispizza.com

100% reccommend!

Formerly Romio's Pizza and the first to offer a HUGE gluten-free menu. RAZZiS have every gluten-free Italian dish you never knew you wanted including focaccia sandwiches, gyros, pizza, pasta, lasagna, ravioli, spaghetti, and desserts.

It's an old-shool, nostalgic, Americanized Italian joint known for their comfort food. Don't eat too much, stomach-aches will ensue.

NOLLIE'S CAFÉ 🌾🌾🌾

ⓘ *Sandwiches and Baked Goods*
Not Dedicated Gluten-Free

📍 **Address:**
1165 Harrison St
Seattle, WA 98109

📞 **(206) 402-6724**

🔗 www.nolliescafe.com

Nollie's Café is a hole-in-the-wall sandwich shop that will make any sandwich with gluten-free bread. They also have several gluten-free homemade treats as well. I really enjoyed eating here when I worked for Amazon, it was never busy and the staff was super friendly.

WAYWARD VEGAN CAFÉ 🌾🌾🌾🌾

ⓘ *Vegan Café*
Not Dedicated Gluten-Free

📍 **Address:**
5253 University Way NE
Seattle, WA 98105

📞 **(206) 524-0204**

🔗 www.waywardvegancafe.com

The name of this restaurant is fitting, since it's in a part of town the attracts a good deal of wayward citizens. Those citizens are most definitely hungry, so they have an entire vegan and gluten-free menu, stocked with breakfast, lunch and dinner dishes.

CUISINE GUIDE

YELLOW DOT CAFÉ

(i) *Sandwich Shop*
Not Dedicated Gluten-Free

📍 **Address:**
301 Westlake Ave N
Seattle, WA 98109

📞 **(206) 381-9200**

🔗 www.yellowdotcafe.com

Yellow Dot Café is a busy little sandwich and soup shop that serves any sandwich on gluten-free bread. They do not have a dedicated grill for warm sandwiches, but if you are not celiac it's a good to-go option.

Seafood

SEASTAR RESTAURANT AND RAW BAR

(i) *Seafood*
Not Dedicated Gluten-Free

📍 **Bellevue:**
205 108th Ave NE
Bellevue, WA 98004

📞 **(425) 456-0010**

📍 **South Lake Union:**
2121 Terry Ave #108
Seattle, WA 98121

📞 **(425) 462-4364**

🔗 www.seastarrestaurant.com

According to Seattle Magazine, Seastar is one of the best seafood restaurants in town. It's definitely a delicious spot, especially in South Lake Union. They have a full gluten-free menu available and gluten-free buns for burgers.

TAYLOR SHELLFISH

ⓘ *Seafood*
Not Dedicated Gluten-Free

📍 **Address:**
1521 Melrose Ave
Seattle, WA 98101

📞 **(206) 501-4321**

🔗 www.taylormelrose.com

If you are eating oysters in Seattle, no matter the restaurant, they are most likely come from Taylor Shellfish Farms. Their main headquarters are up north near Bellingham. Taylor also has a small oyster bar in Capitol Hill (thank goodness) serving strictly fish and daily fish chowders. This is how it works; you choose the (sometimes live) crustacean and they will serve it up for you. Be warned, eating here isn't cheap.

Spanish

HUNGER

ⓘ *Spanish, Dinner and Weekend Brunch*
Not Dedicated Gluten-Free

📍 **Address:**
3601 Fremont Ave N
Seattle, WA 98103

📞 **(206) 402-4854**

🔗 www.hungerseattle.com

Hunger's ambiance is a little too open for my taste. They took over a restaurant space that was built more for the late night bar scene, so if it feels a bit cold, it isn't Hunger's fault. First and foremost the food here is perfectly prepared Spanish/ Morrocan-style. Everything that can be made gluten-free

CUISINE GUIDE

is marked on the menu and if it isn't ask your server. The service is a little spotty, but it is worth the wait, I can't use enough superlatives to explain how good their food is.

TANGO RESTAURANT AND LOUNGE

ⓘ *Spanish and Cuban Fusion*
Not Dedicated Gluten-Free

📍 **Address:**
1100 Pike St
Seattle, WA 98101

📞 **(206) 583-0382**

🔗 www.tangorestaurant.com

Tango has a menu devoted entirely to gluten-free and boy are we thankful for it. This restaurant is more tapa-style, aka small delicious morsels of goodness. That's the technical definition. Little joke. Anyhow, the food is prepared very well and the gluten-free desserts are super decadent.

Sushi

WASABI BISTRO

ⓘ *Sushi*
Not Dedicated Gluten-Free

📍 **Address:**
2311 2nd Ave
Seattle, WA 98121

📞 **(206) 441-6044**

🔗 www.wasabiseattle.com

Sushi is one of my favorite treats, however it's hard to know the little nuances of what has gluten and what does not. Wasabi Bistro takes care of that for you. Their printed menu has an entire gluten-free section with all the rolls that do not contain gluten. Don't let the swanky, upscale décor of this restaurant fool you, they aim to please and are happy to have new customers.

SHIKU SUSHI

(i) *Sushi*
     Not Dedicated Gluten-Free

📍 **Address:**
    5310 Ballard Ave NW
    Seattle, WA 98107

📞 **(206) 588-2151**

🔗 www.shikusushi.com

Shiku Sushi has a trendy vibe and a busy dinner hour. It's dark, attracts a 30-something crowd and all the sushi chefs wear black fedora hats. Their sushi has a certain finesse you can't find anywhere else in Seattle. They do not have a gluten-free menu, but do cater to customers with gluten allergies, just ask your hipster server.

CUISINE GUIDE

Tea

MIRO TEA 🌾🌾🌾🌾🌾

ⓘ *Tea Shop, Crêperie, Desserts*
   Not Dedicated Gluten-Free, but almost!

📍 **Address:**
   5405 Ballard Ave NW
   Seattle, WA 98107

📞 **(206) 782-6832**

🔗 www.mirotea.com

Miro Tea 'crêpes it real' in the most hipster-ish part of Ballard. Serving sweet and savory crêpes, this Tea Haus specializes in 100+ choices of herbal teas and has replaced almost all of their baked goods with gluten-free options for all the allergics out there. I recommend this Cêprerie for remote working and lunching options. See my write up on Miro Tea in our Best-of section.

REMEDY TEAS 🌾🌾🌾

ⓘ *Tea*
   Not Dedicated Gluten-Free

📍 **Address:**
   345 15th Ave E
   Seattle, WA 98112

📞 **(206) 323-4832**

🔗 www.remedyteas.com

Remedy Teas has over 150 organic teas, in fact you can look through their entire catalog of teas and find just the right one for you. Are you tired? Stressed? Needing a detox? They will spell it out for you. If you want a frothy, sweet drink they do that too. You can also order delicious healthy food, they have gluten-free options.

TEAHOUSE KUAN YIN

ⓘ *Tea*
Not Dedicated Gluten-Free

📍 **Address:**
1911 N 45th St
Seattle, WA 98103

📞 **(206) 632-2055**

🔗 www.teahousekuanyin.com

If you want the good stuff, like real Chinese tea, visit Teahouse Kuan Yin. While they are mostly tea, at times they have gluten-free treats to satiate a sweet tooth. Read a book, sip some warm, flavorful tea and relax because you will want to stay awhile here.

Thai

KAOSAMAI THAI RESTAURANT

ⓘ *Thai*
Not Dedicated Gluten-Free

📍 **Address:**
404 N 36th St
Seattle, WA 98103

📞 **(206) 925-9979**

🔗 www.kaosamai.com

Kaosamai is several curries above the rest. Located in a quaint little pink house in Fremont, most of their menu is naturally

CUISINE GUIDE

gluten-free. Kaosamai gets a little creative with their food, which I appreciate. The pumpkin curry, for example is rich and exceptionally flavorful. They also operate a food truck in South Lake Union which is cash only.

May Thai 🌶🌶🌶🌶

(i) *Thai*
Not Dedicated Gluten-Free

📍 **Address:**
1612 N 45th St
Seattle, WA 98103

📞 **(206) 675-0037**

🔗 www.maythaiseattle.com

My top pick for Thai food in Seattle. This restaurant uses the freshest of ingredients and also has all gluten-free dishes marked on their menu. Try their pad thai, I know it's the most "normal" menu item, but May Thai's pad thai is an entirely different animal. I'm not going to say what they do, I don't want to ruin the surprise. Trust me, you will be happy you got it. Best of all the downstairs lounge serves until 2 in the morning.

Siam Thai Cuisine 🌶🌶

(i) *Thai*
Not Dedicated Gluten-Free

📍 **Address:**
1629 Eastlake Ave E
Seattle, WA 98102

📞 **(206) 322-6174**

🔗 www.siamthairestaurants.com

Thai food has quite a few gluten-free options if soy sauce and other sauces containing gluten are not used. Siam Thai has above average thai food, packed with rice noodles, veggies and meat. Check with your server for dishes that are gluten-free.

Vegan/Vegetarian/Raw

CAFE FLORA

(i) *Vegetarian*
     Not Dedicated Gluten-Free

📍 **Address:**
    2901 E Madison St
    Seattle, WA 98112

📞 **(206) 325-9100**

🔗 www.cafeflora.com

Cafe Flora really is about boosting your tummy flora. This restaurant is hands down the best Vegetarian restaurant in Seattle. Most dishes are so well-prepared that you'd never miss the lack of meat. They list what items are available vegan and gluten-free on their menu and carry Maninis Gluten-free Pasta.

CHACO CANYON CAFÉ

(i) *Raw and Vegan Café*
     Not Dedicated Gluten-Free

📍 **University:**   📍 **West Seattle:**
    4757 12th Ave NE   3770 SW Alaska St
    Seattle, WA 98105   Seattle, WA 98126

📞 **(206) 522-6966**   📞 **(206) 937-8732**

🔗 www.chacocanyoncafe.com

For the vegan and raw enthusiast, Chaco Canyon Café serves

up a menu of 90-97% organic sandwiches, salads, bowls and
treats. Everything is vegan and some items are gluten-free.

CYBER DOGS INTERNET CAFÉ 🌾🌾

ⓘ *Vegetarian Hot Dogs*
Not Dedicated Gluten-Free

📍 **Address:**
909 Pike St
Seattle, WA 98101

📞 **(206) 405-3647**

🔗 www.cyber-dogs.com

Cyber Dogs is just silly. They have the silliest brand and an
even sillier menu of vegetarian hot dogs served in any which
way you can think of. Ask and they will make you a silly
gluten-free veggie dog.

PLUM BISTRO 🌾🌾🌾

ⓘ *Raw and Vegan*
Not Dedicated Gluten-Free

📍 **Address:**
1429 12th Ave
Seattle, WA 98122

📞 **(206) 838-5333**

🔗 www.plumbistro.com

If you like creative vegan dishes, this is a 'plum' of a place.
It's always busy here and the food is light, fresh and well-
prepared. Most of the dishes on Plum's menu are made
gluten-free and are marked clearly.

SILENCE-HEART NEST 🌾🌾🌾

ⓘ *Vegetarian, Breakfast and Lunch*
Not Dedicated Gluten-Free

📍 **Address:**
3508 Fremont Pl N
Seattle, WA 98103

📞 **(206) 633-5169**

🔗 www.silenceheartnest.com

Does spiritual intention funneled into vegetarian cuisine make it taste better? Maybe! Silence-Heart Nest is run by a spiritual Krishna-type group in Fremont who serve delicious gluten-free breakfast and lunch in their signature robes. My favorite breakfast dish has to be the eggs benedict, they will substitute gluten-free bread in for this delicious, vegetarian version of a classic.

SUTRA 🌾🌾🌾🌾🌾

ⓘ *Vegetarian, Vegan*
Not Dedicated Gluten-Free

📍 **Address:**
1605 N 45th St
Seattle, WA 98103

📞 **(206) 547-1348**

🔗 www.sutraseattle.com

Sutra has an unforgettable (Portlandia), reservation-only dining experience. Serving two times each evening, you come for a prefix dinner menu of nurtured and named vegetarian dishes. To my delight, when I requested a gluten-free option (when I made a reservation), they did just that. Sutra's food is vegetarian/vegan, but you'd never know it. When I dined there they made lasagna (gluten-free for me) and it was just as good as the real thing.

CUISINE GUIDE

THE JUICY CAFE

ⓘ *Breakfast and Juice Cafe, Vegetarian*
Not Dedicated Gluten-Free

📍 **Address:**
725 Pike St, Fl 2nd
Seattle, WA 98101

📞 **(206) 682-6960**

🔗 www.thejuicycafe.com

The Juicy Cafe has all sorts of healthy menu items from smoothies and raw juices to veggie boxes and gluten-free breakfast bowls. They are located in the Washington State Convention Center, so unless you are checking out Emerald City Comicon or The Northwest Women's Show, you may not find yourself in the vicinity.

THRIVE

ⓘ *Raw, Vegan and Gluten-Free*
Dedicated Gluten-free Facility

📍 **Address:**
1026 NE 65th St
Seattle, WA 98115

📞 **(206) 525-0300**

🔗 www.generationthrive.com

Are you gluten-free, raw, dairy-free, soy-free and vegan? Then Thrive is the place for you. While they may fall short on fattening and inflammatory ingredients, they are absolutely not short on raw, amazing taste. It's one of our favorite places to eat. Try the Buddha Bowl, which has chard, quinoa, dehydrated kale, cashew cream, brown rice, cucumbers, and mushrooms. It is flavored very well and the perfect meal for lunch or dinner. Their mouth watering desserts are based on Jodee Capo's creations of Jodee's Dessert.

CUISINE GUIDE

VEGAN CAKES BY JENNYMAC 🌾🌾🌾

ⓘ *Desserts*
   Not Dedicated Gluten-Free

📍 **Address:**
   4230 2nd Ave NE
   Seattle, WA 98105

📞 **(206) 495-2149**

🔗 www.vegancakesbyjennymac.com

I haven't actually ordered a cake or dessert from Jenny, but I see she does offer gluten-free options. She gets a five star rating and seems to be the place to go if you are allergic to multiple ingredients like egg, soy or sugar.

WAYWARD VEGAN CAFÉ 🌾🌾🌾🌾

ⓘ *Vegan Café*
   Not Dedicated Gluten-Free

📍 **Address:**
   5253 University Way NE
   Seattle, WA 98105

📞 **(206) 524-0204**

🔗 www.waywardvegancafe.com

The name of this restaurant is fitting, since it's in a part of town the attracts a good deal of wayward citizens. They have an entire vegan and gluten-free menu, stocked with breakfast, lunch and dinner dishes. See my write up on Thrive in our Best-of section.

CUISINE GUIDE

Vietnamese

BOL PHO BISTRO ✑✑✑✑

(i) *Vietnamese*
     Not Dedicated Gluten-Free

📍 **Address:**
     918 NE 64th St
     Seattle, WA 98115

📞 **(206) 397-4782**

🔗 www.bolbistro.com

Not all pho is created equal. Most Pho restaurants don't claim
to serve anything of the organic or local variety. Which is
why BOL is better. Everything is organic and made from
sustainable ingredients. The chicken is literally pulled off the
bone for each bowl of soup. Everything at BOL is gluten-free
except the bahm-mi.

TAMARIND TREE ✑✑✑✑

(i) *Vietnamese*
     Not Dedicated Gluten-Free

📍 **Address:**
     1036 S Jackson St
     Seattle, WA 98104

📞 **(206) 860-1404**

🔗 www.tamarindtreerestaurant.com

Chopsticks down, Tamarind Tree is the best Vietnamese food
in Seattle. The ingredients are fresher, the service is better
and most items on the menu are naturally gluten-free. Please
ask your server to clarify if you are unsure of a dish.

LONG PROVINCIAL 🌿🌿🌿🌿

(i) *Vietnamese*
Not Dedicated Gluten-Free

📍 **Address:**
1901 2nd Ave
Seattle, WA 98101

📞 **(206) 443-6266**

🔗 www.longprovincial.com

Long Provincial is Tamarind Tree's sister restaurant. The menu is very similar and offers a plethora of naturally gluten-free dishes. Little secret, they serve the same food as Tamarind Tree and are never too busy to get you in 10 minutes or less. Tamarind Tree has waits as long as an hour and is super busy during dinner hour.

CUISINE GUIDE

INDEX

Symbols

A

B

P

Q

R

S

T

U

V

W

Y

Z

Acknowledgements

To Michael David, thank you for your friendship and partnership. Without you, I would be nowhere.

My gratitude is graciously extended to the businesses of Seattle for catering to diners with gluten allergies. Thank you for going above and beyond and for enthusiastically supporting the making of this dining guide.

To my friends and family who supported me both financially and emotionally, you know who you are. Thank you for being there.

Lastly, to the Universe. While I am not always grateful for the hard life lessons, those experiences have made me the person I am today and for that, I am thankful.

The Guide to Gluten-Free Blog

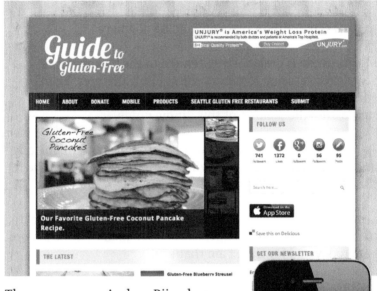

Three years ago, Andrea Bijou began the Guide to Gluten-Free Blog as a resource for people who struggle with gluten allergies. The blog originally began with a few recipes and a Seattle dining guide.

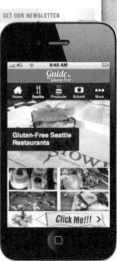

Today, the blog has a shortened dining guide (the extended is in this book), recipes, health articles, new product reviews, spiritual content and other health-related information. For up-to-date gluten-free news and health information, please follow her at www.guidetoglutenfree.com.

About Andrea Bijou

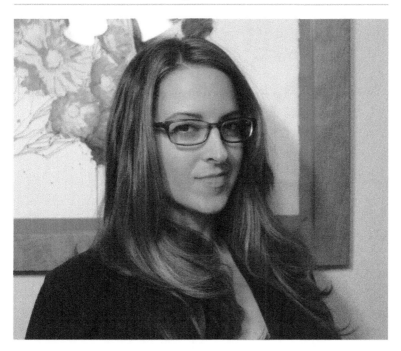

She's dining her way through Seattle, so you can eat just a wee bit easier. Friends and family can attest, Bijou's waistline suffered during the making of this book.

Bijou is a former health and environmental reporter. She had the beats no one wanted and the stories that helped forge our country into a more enlightened way of eating. Now, Bijou brings you a witty and comprehensive look at Seattle's gluten-free foodie scene.

CPSIA information can be obtained at www.ICGtesting.com
Printed in the USA
BVOW11s0619160514

353730BV00001B/3/P